Men

Com

APPROACH

The CommonSense Approach Series

This series of self-help guides from Newleaf provides practical and sound ways to deal with many of life's common complaints.

Each book in the series is written for the layperson, and adopts a commonsense approach to the many questions surrounding a particular topic. It explains what the complaint is, how and why it occurs, and what can be done about it. It includes advice on helping ourselves, and information on where to go for further help. It encourages us to take responsibility for our own health, to be sensible and not always to rely on medical intervention for every ill.

AVAILABLE IN THIS SERIES

Addiction — The CommonSense Approach	Michael Hardiman
Sleep — The CommonSense Approach	Brenda O'Hanlon
Stress — The CommonSense Approach	Brenda O'Hanlon

Menopause

THE CommonSense APPROACH

Ruth Appleby

Newleaf

Newleaf

an imprint of
Gill & Macmillan Ltd
Goldenbridge
Dublin 8
with associated companies throughout the world
© Ruth Appleby 1998
0 7171 2708 7
Index compiled by Helen Litton
Design by Identikit Design Consultants, Dublin
Print origination by Carole Lynch
Printed by The Guernsey Press

This book is typeset in Revivial565 9.5pt on 15pt.

A catalogue record for this book is available
from the British Library.

3 5 4 2

Contents

While the author has made every effort to ensure that the information contained in this book is accurate, it should not be regarded as an alternative to professional medical advice. Readers should consult their general practitioners or physicians if they are concerned about aspects of their own health, and before embarking on any course of treatment. Neither the author, nor the publishers, can accept responsibility for any health problem resulting from using, or discontinuing, any of the drugs described here, or the self-help methods described.

Preface

The menopause is a natural stage in every woman's life. It is my aim to show that every woman can go through this process naturally and gracefully, and come to the realisation of the wisdom we have gained in our lifetime so far. It is a time for vitality and exhilaration, which has become known as the post-menopausal zest! The menopause should not be the end of the road, but the beginning of a new adventure.

Women can experience a new-found confidence in themselves as people. They say in California that 'women have power surges, not hot flushes'. That's confidence! Energy previously spent on rearing children can now be used to achieve new goals. It is a time to seek new careers, to pursue other interesting activities and ambitions. The wisdom, experience and self-confidence gained over the years will far outweigh the 'perceived' loss of youth.

Women resist this stage in life year by year. Book shops are full of books on the menopause, some with beautiful, thin, unwrinkled women on the covers looking about thirty-five, implying that hormone replacement therapy (HRT) or natural remedies will keep them looking young and beautiful 'forever'. What is this fear of growing old? We often hear women complaining that it's not fair that when men's hair goes grey they look 'distinguished', but when a woman's hair goes grey she is supposedly no longer attractive to men.

The process of moving forward and making changes in our lives can be challenging at any time, but the menopause is a time when all our fears and anxieties come to the fore. We may be grieving for our youth, for our reproductive possibilities, and we can think that now our life is over. It's the time of life when we are faced with our own mortality — fear of ageing, fear of death. We may have experienced our parents dying and realise that we are 'the next generation'. Many women will feel less attractive, be depressed, irritable and have mood swings. Maybe your children are leaving home and no longer have need of you and there is a huge void in your lives. Many women feel left on the scrap heap. Yet why should you? Life is moving you forward and you resist it. It is a time for reflection, to look at how much you have done and gained in your life. Give yourself credit for all you have achieved in your life — don't criticise yourself. Women should be confident and, if we approach the menopause with a positive attitude and do not try to resist it, then it can be a time when women come into their power.

Let's look at the menopause from a general health perspective. Health is about adaptability and reaching your potential. Life is constantly changing and flowing. Circumstances change in your life and a healthy response is one of adaptability, overcoming the problem and moving forward. When we are stuck and unable to move forward, the life-force diminishes and we become unbalanced, our health deteriorates and we can develop disease. So a healthy state is one of moving forward with as much ease as possible. It is not one of looking young and attractive forever.

We all aim to pass through the menopause with confidence and serenity. Most women have no problems with the transition, while others may have great difficulty. In this book, we will look at the many options available to women who experience difficulties at this time in their lives. We will look at HRT, and will also consider the many natural and holistic ways of dealing with menopausal symptoms, such as homeopathy, diet, herbal remedies, exercise and various supplements, all of which will alleviate the symptoms of the menopause. Many of the therapies described in these pages can be combined, such as homeopathy with a good diet and plentiful and appropriate exercise.

Acknowledgments

I would like to thank the following: my editor, Eveleen Coyle, for all her help and encouragement; Linda Southgate, for the dietary advice given to me and also for her wisdom; Julie Costello, for her friendship and information on HRT; Patricia Partridge, for her encouragement and friendship; and my partner, Liam McDonnell, without whose support and encouragement this book would never have been finished.

CHAPTER 1

What is Health?

The definition of health in the *Oxford English Dictionary* is 'the state of being well in body or mind'. So what does 'being well' mean?

We could say it means freedom. Freedom from the restrictions of pain or discomfort on the physical level; freedom from fears, anxieties and worries on the emotional level; and freedom from prejudice, egotism and selfishness on the mental level, allowing the mind to concentrate, think clearly, analyse and make rational decisions.

In addition, we can say that it means being adaptable. Life is constantly changing and flowing and we need to move with it. We all have stresses and strains in our lives; our circumstances change from time to time and, if we are 'healthy', we will adapt to these stresses and changes with relative ease and move forward in our lives. When we are stuck, when we can't cope with life and we are unable to adapt and move forward, our health is already beginning to deteriorate. Eventually, even small difficulties that we would normally have coped with easily become a problem. This can happen on any level, either physically, mentally or emotionally.

Fears, inadequacies and feelings of unworthiness all hold us back in life and stunt our growth. This is not a healthy state. If we followed the words of Nelson Mandela, just imagine how our lives would change:

Our deepest fear is not that we are inadequate. Our deepest fear is that we are powerful beyond measure. It is our light, not our darkness, that most frightens us. We ask ourselves: 'Who am I to be brilliant, gorgeous, talented, fabulous?' Actually, who are you not to be? You are a child of God. Your playing small doesn't serve the world. There's nothing enlightened about shrinking so that other people won't feel insecure around you. We are all meant to shine, as children do. We were born to make manifest the glory of God that is within us. It's not just in some of us, it's in everyone. And as we let our own light shine, we unconsciously give other people permission to do the same. As we're liberated from our own fear, our presence automatically liberates others.

If we can achieve a so-called state of 'health', with a freedom on all levels, we can then creatively develop ourselves to the highest potential of our existence. If not, we find ourselves in a 'cramped state', where our overall vision of life can be confined to daily drudgery, and occasioning regrets for those missed opportunities. This occurs more particularly in later years.

Some thoughts from the nineteenth century on how to be healthy are listed below:

- ◆ health makes for long life, efficiency and success
- ◆ eating slowly is time well spent
- ◆ we live not upon what we eat, but upon what we digest
- ◆ physical exercise induces good circulation, sound digestion and mental activity
- ◆ cheerfulness promotes good digestion; it is good to dismiss work, worries and business cares while eating
- ◆ plenty of fresh air makes the fires of life and health burn brightly

- a draught does less harm than foul air
- dust contains the germs of disease
- sunshine should be freely admitted to every home: it is better to have faded carpets than faded cheeks
- work builds up and makes strong the brain; worry wears it out and destroys it
- don't tire the body till it can't be rested
- the human body is a wonderful machine — the more attention it receives, the longer it will last.

These may seem trite, but they are very relevant!

Health is achievable. Freedom is achievable. You are the most important person you know, so if you look at yourself in that way, you must look after yourself as carefully as you would your most prized possession. Interfere with the natural workings of the body as little as possible. Don't always look for a pill to solve a problem. Natural therapies can help. Nourish yourself well in the widest possible sense — exercise, adopt a positive attitude, be fearless and trust in life.

CHAPTER 2

Early Symptoms
of Menopause

It must be stated that most women have no problems at the menopause. Seventy-five to eighty per cent of women experience one or more symptoms, and about thirty per cent have severe symptoms.

The main early symptoms are:

◆ menstrual irregularities
◆ hot flushes and night sweats
◆ dryness of vagina
◆ frequency of urination and incontinence.

Menstrual Irregularities

Irregular periods are usually the first sign that the body is changing. Some women menstruate more frequently than before, others skip periods or find that their periods are more widely spaced apart. Some have ovulation or premenstrual bleeding, which is breakthrough bleeding midway through the cycle; or stop-and-start bleeding at the beginning of the period. Flooding, which is very heavy, and extended bleeding can occur. This in itself will almost certainly lead to anaemia, because the body simply doesn't have time to make up the blood loss before another period arrives. Then you can feel weak, exhausted, worn out, depressed, with headaches, palpitations, etc., and you will blame the menopause for this, when in fact anaemia is the reason.

Heavy or very frequent regular periods, though common, are not normal during the menopause, nor is any sort of vaginal bleeding after the menopause. Always get professional advice about bleeding of this type. Irregular periods do not mean that you can't get pregnant, so it's best to wait until your periods have stopped for two years before you stop using contraception.

Natural ways to help yourself are outlined below:

1 From a dietary point of view, you could increase your intake of foods rich in easily absorbed iron — beef, pork, lamb, organ meats (e.g. liver), poultry, fish, cooked dried beans (e.g. soya or kidney beans), dark-green leafy vegetables (e.g. spinach) and dried fruits. Animal products provide more easily absorbable iron than vegetables.

2 If you need to take an iron supplement, take as directed on the packet. A normal dose is 20–30 mg daily. Large doses of iron supplements may cause stomach upsets and constipation. They can also compete with other minerals and lead to nutritional imbalances. It is not advisable to take tea for half an hour before and after taking iron supplements, as tea stops the absorption of iron.

3 To increase iron absorption, it is important to incorporate vitamin C in your diet, from juices or fruits such as oranges, grapefruits, lemons and kiwis. This can increase iron absorption as much as 30 per cent. If you wish to take a vitamin C supplement, the recommended daily dose is 1,000–3,000 mg.

4 A vitamin B complex, 50 mg daily, also helps with iron assimilation and benefits hormones.

5 Zinc is also important. It promotes a healthy immune system. If you wish to take a supplement, the recommended

daily dose is 15–25 mg. Zinc is found in the following food sources: fish, vegetables, meats, oysters, poultry, seafood and whole grains. Significant quantities of zinc are also found in brewer's yeast, egg yolks, lamb chops, liver, mushrooms, pecan nuts, pumpkin seeds, sardines, seeds, soya lecithin, soya beans and sunflower seeds.

6 Evening Primrose Oil is also beneficial. It contains the highest amount of gamma-linolenic acid (GLA) of any food substance. GLA is an essential fatty acid. The body doesn't manufacture GLA, it must be supplied through the diet. This fatty acid is known to help prevent hardening of the arteries, heart disease, premenstrual syndrome, high blood pressure and female disorders such as cramps, heavy bleeding and hot flushes. Take 500 mg three times daily at the start. After a while, you may be able to reduce to 50 mg twice daily.

Hot Flushes and Night Sweats

Studies show that between fifty and eighty per cent of menopausal women experience hot flushes, which are the body's reaction to the fall in oestrogen levels. When oestrogen levels stabilise, the hot flushes should stop. Women describe a hot flush as heat rising from the upper body to the face. The sensation of a hot flush usually lasts for about three to five minutes. They are likely to happen more frequently after your periods have stopped, and can last for several years. If they are severe, there can also be night sweats, which wake you from sleep. Some women only experience flushes during the day; others only experience night sweats.

Some help for hot flushes has been found in the following.

1 Sage tea or tincture, taken as an infusion, has tonic and hormonal properties. It's good for inflammation and excessive perspiration, and it also has oestrogenic properties.

2 Bioforce Menosan — a tincture of sage.

3 Cucumber drink — liquidise a cucumber and add to one pint of water, store in the fridge, and take one glassful before going to bed.

4 Vitamin C. American tests have shown that vitamin C and bioflavonoid supplements (especially hesperidin) totally relieved hot flushes and other menopausal symptoms in most of the women tested. The testers took daily doses of 1,200 mg of vitamin C and 1,200 mg of hesperidin complex.

5 Vitamin E* — 100 iu to 400 iu daily. You should increase the dose slowly until the flushes cease. (A warning note — 200 iu vitamin E is the maximum dose for people with high blood pressure.) Vitamin E is absorbed better in the presence of fats, so it is better if it is taken at the end of meals.

6 Siberian ginseng, in capsule form, is good for hot flushes, sweats, headaches and palpitations.

7 Potassium — found in bananas and oranges.

8 Homeopathic remedies, such as *Lachesis*, *Graphites*, *Pulsatilla* and *Sulphuric acid*. For hot flushes of sudden onset, use *Amylenum nitrosum*.

9 Regular deep breathing and relaxation when you feel a hot flush coming on.

10 Wear cotton underwear and light clothes.

11 Avoid spicy foods and hot drinks.

12 Avoid hot baths.

13 Stop smoking. Smoking affects the circulation, and intensifies hot flushes and night sweats.

14 Take regular physical exercise. It has been found that women who exercise tend to have fewer hot flushes than those who don't. Exercise improves the circulation, and can make your body more tolerant of temperature changes.

15 Turn your central heating down and keep your rooms well ventilated.

Dryness of Vagina

Some women experience thinning and shrinking of the vaginal walls, loss of elasticity and dryness or itching, which can make intercourse uncomfortable and sometimes painful. This can cause some anxiety in a sexual relationship, as painful intercourse can put a woman off sex and her partner may think she doesn't love him or is no longer attracted to him. Communication, therefore, is very important at this time. But one of the best ways to maintain lubrication of the vagina is to have intercourse, because it increases the blood flow in the vagina. Explain to your partner that you need to take things slowly, and spend more time on foreplay to encourage natural lubrication. Lubricating jelly can also help with discomfort during intercourse.

Some self-help measures that you can take to help all these symptoms are listed below.

1 Vitamin E* — 100 iu to 400 iu per day. Increase the dose slowly until the flushes cease. (A warning note — 200 iu vitamin E is the maximum dose for people with high blood pressure.) Vitamin E is found in the following foods: cold-pressed vegetable oils, whole grains, dark-green leafy vegetables, organ meats, wheat germ, oatmeal and milk.

    In Dr Marilyn Glenville's book *Natural Alternatives to HRT*, she suggests inserting a vitamin E capsule in the vagina every night for six weeks, and then use as needed.
2 Extract of wild Mexican yam, in substances such as Progone Cream (Irish) or Perfect Woman herbal vaginal cream.

Frequency of Urination and Incontinence

Urinary symptoms are very common during the menopause. The urethra can become dry and sore, causing discomfort in passing urine, and there can be frequent and urgent urination even when there is very little urine in the bladder. Some women can experience stress incontinence, which is when urine escapes on coughing, laughing or sometimes just walking.

Things that you can do to help all these symptoms are as follows.

1 Vitamin E* — 100 iu to 400 iu per day. (A warning note — 200 iu vitamin E is the maximum dose for people with high blood pressure.)
2 Extract of wild Mexican yam, in substances such as Progone Cream (Irish) or Perfect Woman herbal vaginal cream, can help.
3 Drink at least eight glasses of water daily to keep the bladder flushed out, especially if you are prone to cystitis.
4 The pelvic floor muscles can be strengthened by alternately tightening and relaxing them as you urinate, so that the stream of urine stops and starts, and stops and starts.
5 If you are overweight, try to lose weight; this will relieve some of the downward pressure on the bladder.
6 Wearing loose cotton underwear will help prevent irritation of the urogenital tract.

The next chapter outlines the symptoms which can develop later in the menopause.

* Vitamin E is always sold in international units (iu).

CHAPTER 3

Later Symptoms of Menopause

The drop in oestrogen that happens at the time of the menopause can cause the following symptoms:

- poor memory and lack of concentration
- insomnia
- panic attacks
- anxiety and depression
- forgetfulness
- loss of libido
- osteoporosis (brittle bones), especially of the hips, lower back and wrists.

Poor Memory and Lack of Concentration

Although most women have no problems during the menopause, during the later stage some women complain of poor memory and lack of concentration. You may forget where you put something, or miss appointments. Some women find they can't make even the simplest decision. This is very distressing for women, and they can often think that they are going senile.

Essential fatty acids aid in the normal functioning and development of the brain, and help in the ability to learn and recall information. These are found in oily fish, such as salmon and mackerel, so include oily fish meals in your diet every week. Supplements thought to be good for the brain include: Gingko Biloba, co-enzyme Q-10, the multi-B vitamin which contains vitamin B1 (thiamine) and vitamin B12, choline, zinc, magnesium and calcium. There is some evidence that these vitamins may aid intellectual symptoms, such as forgetfulness and lack of concentration.

Insomnia

Anxieties and worries can prevent sleep and, when you finally get to sleep, hot flushes can wake you! Your sleep may also be disturbed by having to get up in the night to go to the toilet, and it is common to wake early in the mornings. Women often say that they can put up with the hot flushes, but they can't stand the loss of sleep. This continuous lack of sleep can cause women to become depressed.

The first thing you need to do is to try to get rid of the hot flushes (see the suggestions in Chapter 2). The herbal remedy St John's Wort is helpful for sleeplessness during menopause. It can excite the nervous system if taken on a continual basis, so try taking it for two weeks on and two weeks off. Taking a long walk or some other form of aerobic exercise an hour before bedtime should help the quality of your sleep. Drinking warm milk at bedtime helps too.

Panic Attacks

Some women experience panic attacks. These can be frightening, particularly if you have never had one before. Symptoms can be palpitations, with fear and anxiety for no reason, and panic about being unable to cope in situations where you normally would have had no problem. You feel confused — it is like everything is outside your control. One bad experience may lead to more, and then the fear of an attack alone can bring about another one.

Deep breathing in these situations is invaluable. The Bach Flower remedy Rock Rose can also help.

Anxiety and Depression

Try to overcome anxieties by learning to relax and take deep breaths when you feel anxious or upset. It is easy to be depressed if you are feeling exhausted, with hot flushes, heavy periods and irritability. Don't feel it is all in the mind — share your feelings with your partner and friends.

Essential oils of lavender and chamomile help to relieve anxiety. Use a few drops in the bath, or put some on a handkerchief and inhale it from time to time. You could also put a few drops on the corner of your pillow at night. For tension and anxiety, Bioforce ginsavena and valerian can also help.

Exercise is beneficial to depression. Twenty to thirty minutes of strenuous exercise causes the release of endorphins, which can lift your mood. Start gradually, building up to a more energetic pace after a few weeks. Exercising with a friend will be more fun and will encourage you to continue it. Yoga, relaxation techniques and meditation are also helpful. Great benefit can be found in using such herbs as basil, rosemary and hops, which can be used in cooking, or made into herbal teas. Basil and rosemary are energising and uplifting, giving you a sense of well-being. Use them in the early part of the day when you are looking for more energy. Hops are good for depression too, but they help in a more calming way; as such, they would be used more in the evening.

Keeping blood-sugar levels on an even keel can help avoid highs and lows. Avoiding caffeine helps too, in such substances as coffee, tea, cola and chocolate.

Taking a vitamin B complex supplement daily can help with any symptoms of stress.

Forgetfulness

Forgetfulness is one of the most common symptoms of menopausal women. You may forget where you put something, forget appointments, become confused about things and find making simple decisions difficult.

Keep your brain active by studying something you have an interest in. There are many evening classes available at local colleges. Your brain is like a muscle — the more you use it, the better it becomes. There are a number of nutrients which can boost your brain power, through improving electrical impulses passing through your nervous system. Especially important in maintaining memory are iron, beta carotene and vitamins B1 and B2. These are found in dark green and orange vegetables, liver, nuts and shellfish. Of all the herbs, rosemary is the best memory enhancer, as it stimulates the adrenal cortex.

Loss of Libido

Reaching the menopause is not an end to sexuality, given that for women, procreation and sexuality are separate things. Contrary to the myth that the menopause means women lose interest in sex, many women report that mid-life brings the best sex ever. Post-menopausal women no longer need to worry about contraception, or the risk of unwanted pregnancy. The menopause may cause thinning and drying of the vaginal walls, which results in some discomfort; this can be easily treated, and it does not affect libido. Research shows that women who had a healthy sex life before menopause continue to do so afterwards.

Osteoporosis

Information on osteoporosis and how best to combat it can be found in Chapter 5.

Generally, try some of the advice and remedies described in this book to help yourself. If your symptoms persist, consult professional help.

CHAPTER 4

Menopause

Climacteric

Peri-menopause, menopause and post-menopause are collectively called the climacteric.

The peri-menopausal stage usually starts at around the age of forty-five, and ends between the ages of fifty to fifty-two. We are all individuals, so it is not the same for everybody. In some women, the menopause occurs under the age of forty. This is unusual, and is therefore called premature menopause. We don't know why this occurs, except that it can follow a hysterectomy — with or without the removal of the ovaries — or it may happen if there is a family history of premature menopause. Menopause is when periods have ceased for two years in a woman under fifty, and for one year in a woman over fifty. Post-menopause are the years between the end of a woman's fertility and the end of her life. As women are living longer nowadays, this can amount to thirty years.

The 'menopause' is simply the name given to the time in a woman's life when she stops menstruating. It is effectively the reverse of puberty — the major physical change is that the ovaries gradually stop producing the hormones oestrogen and progesterone. This means that the ovaries stop releasing eggs, periods are no more and the woman can no longer have babies.

Hormones

Hormones are naturally occurring, chemical substances produced by various glands in the body. They circulate in the blood stream and act on other parts of the body. There are many different hormones, with a great variety of functions. Oestrogen and progesterone are the female sex hormones and are produced by the ovaries. The monthly changes in the womb are controlled by these hormones, which women have always made.

A woman's normal monthly cycle starts with the hypothalamus in the brain detecting that you have had a period. It tells the pituitary to send hormones to the ovaries, to get them to start working again. That hormone is FSH, or follicle stimulating hormone. The ovaries start making oestrogen. Oestrogen is the dominant hormone for about ten to twelve days, until ovulation, when that follicle emerges with an egg and releases the egg.

The follicle, now called the corpus luteum, switches over and starts making progesterone. Progesterone is the dominant hormone of the woman's second two weeks of the monthly cycle, making changes in the womb lining that gets the uterus ready for implantation by a fertilised egg. The ovaries make the progesterone for eight to twelve days and then, if no pregnancy occurs, it stops making the hormone, which is the signal for a period. The hypothalamus detects this, and starts the whole cycle all over again.

What happens to these hormones at menopause?

When the time of the change of life arrives, the ovaries gradually diminish in size and function, and production of oestrogen is greatly decreased. It is important to understand that this decrease in oestrogen level at the menopause is normal and occurs in every woman. Many people believe that at this point, a woman's oestrogen production stops. In fact, the oestrogen production in the ovaries diminishes gradually, over a ten- to twelve-year period, before it stops altogether.

We still, however, manufacture oestrogen in the adrenal glands and fat cells — though in smaller quantities — so the drop in oestrogen levels is only relative, not complete, and we continue to produce enough oestrogen to keep us well. The production of progesterone practically ceases at the menopause.

Oestrogen

Oestrogen is the collective name given to describe all natural and artificial chemicals which are able to trigger oestrus, that is the release of an egg in a woman. Oestrogen is not a single hormone like progesterone — it is a group of many different compounds, each with different characteristics and actions.

There are three major kinds of oestrogen made in the human body: oestradiol (the most common and the most potent); oestriol; and oestrone. Oestrogen is mainly produced in the ovaries, although small quantities are secreted from the adrenal glands and the placenta during pregnancy; some is also produced in the fat cells. Oestrogen is needed by the body during pregnancy to ensure that the baby develops properly into a female child. At puberty, oestrogen encourages the development of breasts and the expansion of the uterus. After puberty, oestrogen regulates the menstrual cycle, helps maintain bone mass and keeps blood cholesterol levels in check.

Some oestrogens help to protect against cancer of the breast and reproductive system; foods containing oestrogen-like compounds, called isoflavoids, are found in many soya-based foods, such as tofu, miso, pulses, lentils and rye bread. Some plants (over five thousand known) contain phyto-oestrogens; these are plant-like oestrogens, such as are found in French beans and pomegranates. They bind with oestrogen receptor sites and supply a natural oestrogen to the body.

If there are large quantities of oestrogen in the body, it burns out the ovaries and undermines fertility. An excessive quantity of oestrogen can have the following various effects:

- ◆ it stimulates breast tissue and can lead to fibrocystic breast disease
- ◆ it is the likely cause of thirty per cent of breast cancers
- ◆ it is the only known cause of cancer of the uterus
- ◆ it increases blood clotting
- ◆ it interferes with the thyroid hormone
- ◆ it can cause fluid retention and excess body fat
- ◆ it increases the risks of heart disease and strokes
- ◆ it can cause headaches and loss of libido.

Everyone agrees that no one should be on unopposed oestrogen, that is taking oestrogen alone. The main risk is cancer of the uterus, but some women who have had a hysterectomy and therefore can't get cancer of the uterus are still prescribed unopposed oestrogen and risk all the other side-effects described above.

Natural Oestrogen

If hormones are needed, it is far better to consider using natural hormones, those which are chemically identical to the hormones produced by your own body. If a woman needs a little extra oestrogen for a short while, natural oestrogens such as oestriol are far safer than others, such as oestrone or oestradiol.

If you are taking oestrogen, you may need to reduce the dose after adding progesterone; otherwise you may experience oestrogen side-effects.

Progesterone

Progesterone protects the body from the side-effects of oestrogen. The effects of progesterone as a hormone are vastly different from any other hormone. The job of other hormones in the body is to stimulate some reaction in another part of the body. Their work is then finished, and they go to the liver and are excreted in the bile. A major function of progesterone is to help the body produce and regulate certain other steroid hormones, including cortisol, aldosterone, oestrogen and testosterone. So, progesterone is a precursor to a whole range of other hormones, as well as being a hormone on its own.

When you are under stress, either from some trauma, or surgery or an accident, or any other stress in life, your body makes cortisone. This is the appropriate response to stress, but if you are lacking in progesterone, your body has difficulty in manufacturing this much needed stress reliever.

Other intrinsic effects of progesterone on the body are described below. It:

- helps the body to burn fat for energy
- is a skin moisturiser
- is good for scalp hair
- is a mild antidepressant and a natural diuretic
- restores libido
- normalises blood clotting
- normalises blood sugar, zinc and copper levels
- protects against endometrial and breast cancers
- protects against fibrocystic breast disease
- stimulates osteoblasts to make new bones
- is a precursor of cortisone.

It's a great hormone!

During pregnancy, the body produces very large quantities of progesterone and this helps the womb hold the foetus safely until the baby is born. Midwives throughout history have been using wild Mexican yam (*Dioscorea villosa*), a plant that grows throughout Central America and which contains significant concentrations of diosgenin — one of nature's finest sources of natural progesterone — to treat breakthrough bleeding during pregnancy and to prevent threatened miscarriages.

Synthetic progesterone, also called progestins or pro-gestogens, like natural progesterone, can help maintain or sustain the human secretory endometrium, but it is not capable of the wide range of biological activity that natural progesterone performs. Progestins aggravate conditions linked to inadequate progesterone. When a woman takes progestin, her body becomes confused, and produces less natural progesterone; this can cause symptoms such as fluid retention. Progestins aggravate PMS symptoms, can cause breast cancer and hirsutism, while natural progesterone counters both. Progestins can also cause increased blood pressure, depression, weight gain, insomnia, decreased sex drive, hair loss, nausea and dizziness.

Hormonal imbalance in younger women

Dr John Lee, the well-known expert on natural progesterone, has studied problems specific to women, including menopausal problems such as osteoporosis, over a number of years. During the course of his work, Dr Lee asked himself these questions: 'Why should HRT ever be needed? Did mother nature make a mistake in women? Is there a design flaw? Why is this happening?' He noticed that in Third World countries, illnesses such as fibrocystic breast disease, osteoporosis, cancers, premenstrual syndrome and menopausal symptoms don't happen very often — they happen mainly in industrialised countries.

Lee also noticed that there are no historical references to osteoporosis. Osteoporosis is a new phenomenon. It used to develop around menopause, now it is starting at the age of thirty-five. He realised that something was going wrong — and it wasn't mother nature. He examined the bones of women that had been dug up in England from the seventeenth and eighteenth centuries, and found that those bones were stronger than the bones of women in England today. Again, he asked himself the question 'What is happening?'

Dr Lee discussed this with Dr Jerilynn Prior, chief endocrinologist at the University of British Columbia in Vancouver, who was doing tests on women athletes who were fit and healthy, but whose periods had stopped due to heavy strenuous training. What Dr Prior and her colleagues discovered was that a large number of menstruating women are no longer ovulating long before the menopause. Dr Prior published a paper describing how some women in heavy training were developing osteoporosis. She checked their progesterone and oestrogen levels, and thought she would find the cause of the osteoporosis as being lowered oestrogen levels. She found, however, that their oestrogen levels stayed up while their progesterone levels went down. So, it seemed that it was not the lack of oestrogen, but the decline in progesterone levels that caused the osteoporosis.

Dr Prior then decided to test non-athletic women whose body fat levels were normal. She found that the same thing happened — that at about the ages of thirty-three to thirty-five, their progesterone levels were also declining. What was causing this?

At the same time, animal scientists have noticed that the alligators have been dying in Florida, and that seagulls, foxes, frogs, turtles, etc. are not reproducing as they used to. They found a common feature in the females of these animals — that the ovaries' follicles, the ones that produce the eggs, are all burned out. Something is stimulating the overuse of the follicles, which burns them out. The same has been seen in women. The average woman is born with 300,000 follicles, which are meant to last from around the age of fourteen to fifty-four, but now they are being used up by the time the women are in their thirties. In male animals, it has been seen that the sperm are not maturing, and sperm counts are going down. In men too, there has been a twenty-five to thirty per cent drop in sperm count over the last twenty-five years.

Dr Lee says that the cause seems to stem from an increase of oestrogen in our bodies, coming from xenoestrogens. The word xeno means 'strange' or 'foreign'. The animals mentioned above are exposed to petrochemical by-products, by-products of insecticides, by-products of herbicides, by-products of plastic production, the PCBs and the polymers. These chemicals, which are sprayed on our grain and vegetables including the foodstuffs fed to the animals whose meat we eat, are fat soluble. They need to be fat based, so that the insects feeding on these plants will be killed. But these chemicals remain in our food and in the meat that we eat. We accumulate these toxins in the fat of our bodies over the years. People whose diet is more plant and vegetable based have a better chance of limiting their intake of these chemicals, because plants tend to have less fat than animals.

What is happening is that these chemicals are mimicking the oestrogens in the body, acting exactly like a very potent oestrogen in stimulating the follicles to burn themselves out; women then become deficient in progesterone much earlier than before. They can do this because all these xenoestrogens have a phenol ring in common with the oestrogen molecule as part of their chemical structure.

Keeping the balance of oestrogen and progesterone

The oestrogens and progesterone in a woman's body must balance each other for her to stay healthy. If we are absorbing many xenoestrogens into the body, and if the body is deprived of its required amount of progesterone, the production of the other related hormones can be severely unbalanced; we can then end up with an excess of oestrogen in the body. Taking natural progesterone doesn't create an excess of these other hormones. In fact, it acts as a normaliser, by helping to decrease any excess or correct any deficiency.

Am I deficient in progesterone?

The sure way for a women to know whether she is deficient in progesterone is to have a low serum progesterone test done between days eighteen and twenty-six of her menstrual cycle. This test can be organised by her doctor. A normal serum progesterone level after ovulation is approximately 7-28 picograms. If you don't ovulate, your serum progesterone level will tend to be about 0.3 picograms. (One picogram equals one trillionth of a gram.)

Natural plant-derived progesterone

Dr Lee found that when he gave his patients, who were not taking oestrogen, a natural plant-derived form of progesterone, along with recommendations for dietary and lifestyle changes, the bone loss levelled out and their bone mass increased. The progesterone had stimulated the osteoblasts to make new bones. He believes that the natural, plant-derived form of pro-gesterone, along with recommendations for dietary and lifestyle changes, can not only stop osteoporosis but actually reverse it, even in women aged seventy.

Lee then examined his patients who were taking oestrogen, and found that oestrogen alone does not increase your bone density — it doesn't build new bones. The decline of bone density is slowed down when you take oestrogen, but it doesn't reverse the bone loss. So he gave these patients progesterone as well, and their bone density improved. Dr Lee found that people who had poor bones to begin with gained a considerable percentage more bone mineral density than those people whose bones were fairly good at the outset. In the latter case, there was only a slight gain, as you would expect, just enough to maintain the bones.

His patients recorded other improvements when taking progesterone, such as improvements in fibrocystic breast disease, in hypothyroid condition, in water retention, in high blood pressure and in thinning hair. If you are on thyroid supplements, you should get a test within three months of starting to use progesterone, as you may need to reduce the medication.

How to use plant-derived natural progesterone

After much experimentation with different ways of administering progesterone, the safest and most efficient way of administering it seems to be through the skin, by means of a cream. Using the cream as against an oral preparation, it can enter the bloodstream directly, bypassing breakdown by the liver, where up to seventy per cent is metabolised and excreted prior to yielding any benefit. Therefore a much smaller amount of progesterone is needed in cream form. The cream is applied once or twice daily to the skin, which readily absorbs it; it is then distributed throughout the body.

The cream can be applied to any part of your body, but it is recommended to apply it to the largest possible areas of relatively thin skin, such as the inner arms and thighs, the face and neck, the upper chest and the abdomen. Rotating various skin sites daily will help with maximum absorption. If you are severely progesterone deficient, the body fat layers absorb it first. Then, as the fatty tissues become saturated, there is an increase in blood levels of progesterone, and a stronger physiological effect.

What quantity to use?

As to the question of how much of the progesterone creams to use, everybody is different and quantities vary according to individual needs. If you suffer from premenstrual syndrome, the natural progesterone cream is used for two weeks, starting from day fifteen of the cycle. The dose is ⅛ teaspoon twice daily, gradually increasing the amount of cream to ½ teaspoon twice daily in the week before the next period starts. If you are menopausal, it is recommended that you start using the cream on around day eight of a calendar month, using ¼ teaspoon twice daily up to day twenty-one, then increasing to ½ teaspoon twice daily from day twenty-two to the end of a month. Then don't use any creams for a week, and repeat the process.

In the case of using natural progesterone cream for mild osteoporosis, or for the prevention of osteoporosis, it is recommended to use approximately half a jar over a month, skipping the first seven days. This is slightly less than ¼ teaspoon daily. In the case of severe osteoporosis, a full 2 oz/59 ml jar or more should be used, skipping the first seven days as before.

You can adjust the amounts to your own needs. As time goes by and symptoms begin to decrease, try gradually using less of the natural progesterone cream each month. If symptoms return, use the cream as before, and again try to use less and less until it is no longer needed. Use the cream on an 'as needed' basis.

Creams available on the market

There are many of these creams on the market, such as Natragest, Pro-Gest, Progone and Perfect Woman. They contain extracts of wild Mexican yam, which contains significant concentrations of diosgenin, one of nature's finest sources of natural progesterone.

Natragest, from Broadmoor Laboratories, California, is a four per cent natural progesterone cream, from wild Mexican yam, and is available from The Natural Healing Rooms in Cork. Pro-Gest is a three per cent natural progesterone cream, from wild Mexican yam, and is available from The Nutrition Centre in Donegal. Progone is available from Halmont Ltd in Bray, Co. Wicklow. Perfect Woman is available from most health food stores. (For addresses and contact numbers for these sources of natural progesterone, see Useful Addresses.)

I have mentioned Dr Lee's 'oestrogen dominance' theory because it is very much the popular idea at the moment. Dr Lee makes the whole issue sound believable and simple, and I would like to think he is right. But, firstly, there seem to be some queries about how 'natural' the creams are and the processes they go through. Secondly, there is the question of regulating the doses. Because not everyone absorbs progesterone in the same way, who is to say how much progesterone is actually being absorbed by the body, and what happens if we absorb an excess of natural progesterone in the body?

We are told that women should not experience any side effects from the creams, but a number of practitioners are reporting some. In the 'What Doctors Don't Tell You' publication *Guide to the Menopause*, they say: 'Alternative practitioner Marilyn Glenville has had numerous women who have come to her, suffering from a range of problems — bleeding, extreme breast tenderness, terrible PMT-like symptoms — which they claim began after using rub-on cream. One woman developed severe hot flushes after stopping the cream, when she didn't have them before she started using it.' A number of people I know who have been using the creams have reported only benefits in their physical symptoms, and a definite feeling of well-being in themselves. So, the results are confusing.

Much more research needs to be done on this treatment, and I think we need to see the results of many more years of use to truly evaluate these creams. It doesn't seem to be the miracle cure we all hoped for, yet many people are finding be-nefits from it. If the creams are used sensibly and treated with respect, I don't think any harm can come from using them. Obviously, if you suffer any side effects you should stop using the cream immediately.

Remember always that a sensible diet through the menopause is your best route to balance and a healthy body.

CHAPTER 5

Osteoporosis

Bones are living tissue, like your skin or hair. If you break a bone and it is put in plaster, it will heal. Bones are constantly being made, unmade and then made again. When one hundred per cent of the bones have been renewed, this is called the turnover time. Osteoplasts will dissolve away little pockets of bone where the bone is too old, and the osteoblasts come behind them and make new bones. Turnover time for long bones, like the femur or the arm bones, is ten to fourteen years, but for the spine, heels etc. — which are not as tough as the long bones — it only takes two to four years. So, in that time you have entirely new bones.

Bones are comprised of fibres of collagen, which provide elasticity, and calcium, which provides strength. In the ageing process, bones tend to lose both collagen and calcium.

Osteoporosis is diagnosed when the bone loss becomes too great, and the bones become honeycombed, brittle and prone to fractures. The problem is not just caused by lack of calcium in the diet, but also because the bone stops accepting calcium from the blood. Our reserves of calcium are stored in bone tissue, which is added to or taken from as needed to maintain a balance of calcium in the blood. When it is in balance, it helps the heart and brain to function well. When it is deficient in the blood, you can get cramps in the muscles and an irregular pulse rate. Long-term calcium loss is the main cause of low bone density. Our modern, fast pace of life can make it very difficult for us to keep everything in balance.

Ageing is a main cause. Reduced levels of progesterone also seems to be a factor. Other factors are heredity, stress, lack of exercise, eating highly processed, over-refined food, drinking alcohol and smoking.

The types of people most prone to osteoporosis are:

◆ thin
◆ small boned
◆ fair skinned
◆ those who have had their ovaries removed before the age of forty-five
◆ childless
◆ those who have been confined to bed for an extended time
◆ those who are diabetic or hypoglycaemic
◆ lactose intolerant
◆ people who have an underactive thyroid
◆ people who lead a sedentary life
◆ those who avoid dairy products
◆ smokers
◆ long-term dieters
◆ long-term steroids users.

HRT (hormone replacement therapy) is the most popular preventive medicine for osteoporosis. However, research has shown that you need to take HRT for at least seven years for it to have any long-term protective effect on bone mineral. Once women stop HRT, bone loss accelerates rapidly, to the point where, some years later, their bone density loss would be very little less — around three per cent — than those who were never treated with HRT. So, it would seem, to get long-term benefit from HRT for osteoporosis, you would need to take it from the beginning of menopause for the rest of your life. This doesn't seem like a good idea, since it is well established that

HRT increases a woman's risk of breast and endometrial cancers, and long-term use of it would multiply this risk.

There are a number of things you can do to keep your bones healthy and help prevent osteoporosis.

Exercise

Weight-bearing exercises maintain strong healthy bones, therefore protecting you against osteoporosis. Exercise stimulates bones to thicken. As muscles are exercised and strain and contract, bone responds by building denser tissue. So exercise creates calcium in the bones. Exercise also keeps your joints flexible, helps to keep your weight down, boosts your immune system and improves balance and co-ordination. Regular exercise makes you feel good, beats stress and fatigue and helps you to sleep better. It's important to keep active, because calcium drains away from the bones while you rest.

Exercise needs to be incorporated into your life before the problems occur, but it is never too late to begin. If you are only starting to exercise now and are unfit, introduce exercise gently into your life, with walking, swimming, yoga, t'ai chi, dancing, gardening, etc. Avoid carrying heavy loads. Exercise also improves heart and lung function, which in turn helps to protect against coronary heart disease.

Vitamins and Minerals

Calcium

We need calcium in the body at menopause to help with muscle contractions (cramps), nerve impulses, sleeplessness, nervousness and tingling in the arms. At menopause, there is a marked increase in calcium in the urine. Perhaps what we should do is prevent its excretion from the body, rather than continually try to supplement it with more. However, the recommended daily dose of calcium for menopausal women is

500 mg. Excessive calcium can increase the risk of kidney stones, so you need to balance calcium intake with vitamin D and magnesium. Take supplements at night time, the time of greatest bone loss, because as noted above, calcium drains away from the bones while you rest.

Vitamins and minerals that help you hold on to calcium in the body are as follows:

- calcium (500 mg)
- vitamin D (without vitamin D, calcium cannot be absorbed); the recommended dose is 200 iu daily; if you take too high a dose of vitamin D, it can actually extract calcium from bone
- magnesium (250 mg, but not after meals, as magnesium neutralises stomach acidity)
- phosphorus (250 mg; people are not often deficient in phosphorus or vitamin K)
- vitamin K (250 mg)
- manganese (2.5-7 mg)
- zinc (10 mg)
- vitamin B6 (50 mg)
- vitamin C (1,000–3,000 mg)
- boron (3 mg).

All the doses stated are per day.

Substances that leach out and encourage the excretion of calcium from the body are:

- red meat
- protein
- salt
- coffee.

It is therefore important to avoid these.

Sources of calcium, bearing in mind that only twenty per cent of calcium in the diet is absorbed by the body:

- seaweed
- kelp (one of the highest forms of calcium available)
- dairy products (don't depend on dairy products for your total intake of calcium from your diet; cow's milk products also contain a level of phosphorus high enough to interfere with calcium uptake)
- canned fish
- nuts and seeds (sesame seeds are particularly good)
- soya and soya products (tofu)
- green vegetables, such as cabbage and broccoli
- dried beans
- figs
- apricots
- black treacle
- whole grains
- pulses.

Calcium is made less available by eating the following:

- rhubarb
- spinach (oxalic acid)
- outer husks of grains (phytic acid) e.g. brown rice
- a high fat diet
- chocolate.

Some calcium supplements that are available are listed below:

- Floradix Calcium
- Bioforce Urticalcin
- CalMag

- Ostron by Lifeplan (specifically for osteoporosis)
- Nature's Own Calcium.

Try one brand. If it doesn't help after a month, try another.

Magnesium

Some researchers believe that magnesium deficiency, rather than calcium deficiency, is responsible for osteoporosis. Magnesium works with calcium (usually two parts calcium to one part magnesium).

Sources of magnesium:

- green vegetables — the greener the better
- sesame seeds
- soya beans
- nuts, particularly cashew, almonds, brazil, peanuts
- Brewer's yeast
- figs
- apricots.

Some magnesium supplements that are available are listed below:

- Sona Magnesium
- CalMag
- Magnesium OK
- Nature's Own Magnesium.

Boron

Boron is a new mineral, which was only discovered as recently as 1980. There is evidence that this mineral prevents calcium loss and bone de-mineralisation. It activates oestrogen and vitamin D. We only need 3 mg daily, but its function is vital.

Sources of boron are:

◆ vegetables
◆ dairy products
◆ fish
◆ meat
◆ soya beans
◆ prunes
◆ raisins
◆ almonds.

Some boron supplements that are available are:

◆ Boron Tablets
◆ Confiance
◆ Menopace
◆ Ostron by Lifeplan.

Try one brand. If it doesn't help after a month, try another.

Essential Fatty Acids

Two essential fatty acids, gamma-linolenic acid (GLA) and eicosapentaenoic acid (EPA), have been shown to improve calcium balance and bone mineral content. We get GLA in Evening Primrose oil and EPA in fish oils. The quantity to take is usually two parts or more Evening Primrose oil to one part fish oil.

Some essential fatty acid supplements that are available are:

◆ Gamma Marine
◆ Efamol Marine.

Some further advice is outlined below.

Natural Plant-derived Progesterone

Dr Lee recommends the use of a natural plant-derived form of progesterone, which stimulates the osteoblasts to make new bones. He believes the natural plant-derived form of progesterone, along with recommendations for dietary and lifestyle changes, can not only stop osteoporosis but actually reverse it, even in women aged seventy. The most efficient way of administering it seems to be through the skin, by means of a cream.

There are many of these creams on the market, such as Natragest, Pro-Gest, Progone and Perfect Woman. They contain extract of wild Mexican yam, which itself contains significant concentrations of diosgenin, one of nature's finest sources of natural progesterone.

Stop Smoking

Smoking can contribute to osteoporosis. Studies have shown that stopping smoking reduced the risk of osteoporotic fractures.

Get Rid of Your Aluminium Saucepans!

Aluminium can inhibit the parathyroid gland, also leading to osteoporosis.

CHAPTER 6

Diet and Exercise for Good Health During Menopause

How a woman copes physically during the menopause is determined by the body's ability to ride the huge hormonal changes that are sweeping through the system at this stage. The best way to help yourself through the menopause is to be in good shape.

Diet

The body makes hormones from foods, so it makes sense to alter your diet to make allowances for changing hormones in your body. Diet has a direct influence on hormonal balance. Some foods contain specific vitamins which are necessary for hormonal balance, while others are rich in substances that are similar to hormones.

Our food needs are also declining at this time. We should eat less, and eat unrefined food, high in fibre, low in sugar and fats.

Unrefined Foods (Unprocessed, Organic)

Food can be stressful to the body, and we need to make it as easy as possible for the body to process it. This means that the food we eat should be free from chemicals and hormones. Nowadays, there is also increasing irradiation and genetic engineering of our foods. If we look back to fifty years ago, the food choices were fewer, but there was much higher purity of food. In addition, the body didn't have to deal with the toxins and the stresses of the highly refined foods that we eat today.

Put as few chemicals into the body as possible, by choosing unrefined foods. These are foods that have been tampered with as little as possible, e.g. wheat grain. When it is partly processed to produce brown flour, it is made into a brown loaf. When it is processed even more, it is made into white flour and then into a white loaf. So, the more the grain is processed and refined, the further and further away it becomes from the original grain. A grain of wheat would grow if you put it into the ground. Foods that have been tampered with don't have a life-force — they could be categorised as 'dead' food. A lot of convenience food comes into this category.

Try to eat organic food as much as possible, for the same reason. It is easier now to get organic vegetables, fruit, meat, poultry and dairy produce.

Increase Fibre Intake

A lot of our illnesses come from the bowels. A healthy body processes food quickly, takes out the nutrients it needs and eliminates the waste through the bowels. Fibre in the diet helps this process. A lot of the fibre recommended contains the nutrients needed for a healthy body. Bran is not always the most effective way to increase fibre. This is because it is coarse and abrasive, and in some cases can cause blockages. Too much bran can take out some of the nutrients that we need — it acts like blotting paper. Linseeds are better, in that they are gentler on the system.

Use wholemeal flour, bread, potatoes, pasta, brown rice, peas, beans, lentils and vegetables. Also dried fruit and unsalted nuts.

Lower Sugar Intake

When the sugar cane is processed, the best part of it, the molasses, is taken off. This has all the iron, vitamins and minerals in it. It used to be fed to cattle; now it is sold in health food shops as an aid for sleep and arthritis, and as a supplement. When you process it further, you end up with white sugar. All the nourishing things have been taken out by this stage.

Sugar is one of the most addictive foods. People think that they need sugar for energy, but in fact carbohydrate will give you better energy, as it provides a slow release of energy, unlike sugar, which gives you the swings of high and low energy. There are hidden sugars in a lot of foods, like baked beans, soups, tins of sweet corn, etc. Our palate has come to demand sweet things.

Try to cut down on cakes and biscuits. Eat fresh fruit rather than tinned. Watch breakfast cereals for hidden sugars — eat porridge and sugar-free muesli. You can also obtain jams with no added sugar. Watch out for sugar in drinks too.

Lower Fat Intake

Lower your fat intake, especially from animal sources, such as meats and dairy products — cheeses and full-fat milk. The exception to the rule would be fatty fish, such as mackerel, herrings, salmon and sardines, as these contain EFAs (essential fatty acids). In order to lower your fat intake, it is important to cut down on crisps, chocolate, cakes and biscuits.

Dietary Do's and Don'ts

Oils and spreads Use polyunsaturated and unhydrogenated spreads. These help to lower the fats and are good for the heart. Use olive oil, sunflower oil/spread.

Saturated fats Cut down on saturated fats, i.e. animal fats, butter.

Cheese Eat lower fat cheese, e.g. Edam, which is lower in fat than cheddar.

Milk Use skimmed, or semi-skimmed, milk, which has as much calcium as full fat.

Meat Cut down on red meat — it's high in hidden fat.

Salt

It is important to cut down on the quantity of salt you eat. Reduce the amount of salt you use in cooking (flavour with lemon, herbs, spices and mustard instead). Look for 'no added salt' on labels. It is also essential to watch out for salty snacks, e.g. crisps and salted nuts. Make home-cooked soups — packet and tinned soups contain salt. Beware of salt substitutes, as they are not always as low in salt as you would expect. When using salt, use sea salt — it contains valuable minerals, especially iodine, which is good for the thyroid. It has no added chemicals, and you don't need to use as much.

Water

Increase your water intake. You should be drinking four pints of water every day.

Hormone-Like Foods

Foods that fall into the category of helping to cushion the body from the adjustments it makes during menopause are: carrots, ripe bananas, apples, celery, broccoli, leafy greens, cucumber, all berries, papaya, sprouted seeds, linseed, soya flour/products, walnuts and avocado. (These all have natural oestrogen.)

Also use kelp, liquorice, Siberian ginseng (good for loss of libido), Evening Primrose oil (two to three tablets at night), Royal Jelly and alfalfa.

Substances to Avoid

There are particularly adverse foods and drinks which you should take special care to avoid. These include: caffeine, dairy products, fats, fries, junk food, red meat, sugar and fizzy drinks. (Fats and sugars slow down oestrogen production.)

When we are feeling low, we all tend to eat junk food, and then feel worse afterwards — and then feel guilty! Don't be hard on yourself, allow yourself a 'bad' day, enjoy it, and then go back to eating better the next day.

Exercise

The human body is designed for muscular activity, to be moved and exercised, and does not function to its potential or maintain itself properly without exercise. A full range of movements of all parts of the body every day is needed to keep your physical body fit. Regular exercise brings about marked physiological changes and improvement in normal body functioning. It increases muscle strength and creates calcium, thereby building strong bones. Exercise also keeps your joints flexible, helps to keep your weight down, boosts your immune system and improves balance and co-ordination.

Exercise is also good for the mind. It has been shown that exercise can reduce tension and anxiety and, in some cases, depression, by promoting the release of hormone-like sub-stances — including adrenaline and noradrenaline — that affect the emotions. Regular exercise enhances clarity of mind, makes you feel good, helps you to relax, beat stress and fatigue and encourages more restful sleep. Exercise also improves heart and lung function. Maybe this is an opportunity for you now to look at the amount of exercise you are taking, and if you have been a couch potato for years, then this is the time to get up and move that body!

A Gentle Introduction

If you are unfit and have not been taking any form of regular exercise for years, the first thing you should do is check with your doctor before starting on a simple exercise programme. Then you should introduce exercise gently into your daily routine, with aerobic movements such as walking, swimming and/or cycling. Aerobic exercise improves the functioning of the heart, lowers cholesterol and increases noradrenaline, which improves your well-being. It also helps your body to burn fat and keeps you trim.

Walking is an excellent aerobic exercise, as you can walk at your own pace in the fresh air and, after a week or so of walking for about a quarter of an hour a day, you will find that you are able to increase the length and pace of your daily walk. If you use the bus, it's a good idea to get off a couple of stops earlier and walk the rest of the way. Another sensible thing you could do is to use the stairs instead of the lift, or cycle to work. Cycling can relieve anxiety, stress and depression, partly due to the physical exercise, but also because of the simple pleasure of riding. Swimming is also an excellent aerobic exercise, being good for joint mobility and the lungs. If you persevere with exercise and do a little every day, you will soon feel that your body is more alive, you will have more energy and you will find you can relax more easily and sleep better.

Restoring the Balance

Yoga is excellent for flexibility, strength and body awareness. Hatha yoga is the form best known in the West, and the exercises are practised for their overall improvement to the health of the nervous system, glands and vital organs. The word hatha comes from *ha*, meaning 'sun' and *tha*, meaning 'moon'. It is the balance between night and day, dark and light, and when you practise yoga you are trying to get into that balanced state.

During menopause, we become slightly out of balance. Some of the problems are physical, but a lot of them are mental and emotional difficulties that need to be dealt with, and practising yoga is an ideal solution. You are exercising all parts of the body; in addition, yoga also improves your emotional and mental states. It promotes tranquillity, and combats tension and anxiety. The combination of stretching movements, mental relaxation and deep breathing addresses all aspects of the person, and can help deal effectively with the menopausal transition. It is not just a physical regime! It is well worth practising.

T'ai chi is also about balance and balancing energy. *Chi* means 'energy', and t'ai chi is the ability to move the energy around the body. When people think of t'ai chi, what may come to mind is the image of people in China doing these wonderful relaxing exercises in parks in the early mornings. T'ai chi is indeed relaxing, but it also strengthens the body, both physically and mentally, teaches you correct body alignment and improves the circulation.

Dancing is also about balance and is great exercise, with a good range of movements. It's also great fun. So, if you only find yourself dancing after too many drinks at a wedding or at special dinners at Christmas time, then maybe it is time to try it again. Many women are finding Arab dancing, or belly dancing, great fun. The dance is based on movements of the pelvis and spine. It tones up your hips and waist, and gives your abdominal organs an internal massage! It is also a great confidence booster, as Arab dancing actually celebrates women's hips and bottoms, so whatever your size you will gain a great sense of pride in yourself.

Gardening is about balancing nature, observing nature and patience! While it is not as effective as aerobic exercise, where there is a prolonged increase in heart rate, it still keeps you out in the fresh air and moving around.

It has all to do with balance. Some people can become psychologically addicted to exercise and feel compelled to go to the gym every day. This is an imbalance, and can be detrimental to health. When you over-train, you can get mood swings and have difficulties with sleep and your appetite. It can also affect your immune system, making you more susceptible to colds. If you think you are over-training and have become addicted to exercise, you should seek medical help.

The most important aspect of all exercise is that you *enjoy* it!

CHAPTER 7

Stress and Relaxation

Many people these days say they cannot relax. They are on the go all day long, either trying to balance a career with running a home, or working at home and caring for children. Some women say they feel like a taxi service, bringing children to and from school and to extracurricular activities like ballet, hockey, swimming, etc. At the end of the day, they still can't relax because there is always something more to be done. If you spend your life chasing your tail, you will just end up feeling irritable and resentful.

Focus on the Present

It may be true that 'a woman's work is never done', but if you prioritise the things you have to do today and get them done, you can then leave the rest to tomorrow, knowing that you have achieved what you set out to do today. Tomorrow is another day, and if you prioritise on a daily basis you will find that you have more control over your time and that you are achieving what you set out to do each day. In fact, what really happens is that you are concentrating on today, really focusing one hundred per cent on what you have to do today and not criticising yourself for what you didn't do yesterday, or last week, or worrying about all you have to do tomorrow, or next month.

Don't waste time and energy dwelling on past mistakes. Stop blaming yourself when things go wrong. No one is perfect and everyone makes mistakes, so accept that you did the best you could in the circumstances, learn from it and then let it go. Worrying about the future is futile also, as we don't know what the next moment might bring — so why waste precious time worrying about what will happen? This also takes as much energy from you as dwelling on the past.

Then give yourself time to relax, and don't be afraid of the feelings that occur. Experience them and face them head on and then try to understand them. You will then have a better chance of doing something about them.

Relaxation Techniques

Almost all muscle relaxation techniques involve deep breathing. Yoga and relaxation techniques, such as deep breathing and meditation, can promote tranquillity and combat stress, anxiety and tension. Most of us don't breathe properly, and use only a third of our lung capacity: we only use the upper part of the chest, and so deprive the body of valuable oxygen. Try to breathe more deeply and more slowly; apart from improving the function of your lungs, it will relax you completely.

It has also been found that women who meditated had fewer problems during menopause. The meditation can be very simple. Sit or lie somewhere comfortably and just concentrate on your breathing, thinking of nothing else and breathing deeply all the time. If thoughts come into your mind, just go back to concentrating on your breathing. Or, instead of concentrating on your breathing, you can imagine yourself somewhere you have been happy, such as strolling along a beach, on holiday or walking in a park listening to the birds. Again, if you find thoughts coming into your mind, simply go back to concentrating on where you were in your happy place. Do this for five minutes, and you will find yourself a lot calmer afterwards.

Another relaxation technique is 'Observe the Five Senses' exercise:

> *Touch*
> Sit and be aware of your body. Feel each part.
> *Taste*
> Be aware of your taste. What can you taste now?
> *Smell*
> Become aware of any odours around you.
> *Sight*
> Be aware of your sight, but don't hold your gaze on anything in particular.
> *Hearing*
> Try to hear the softest sounds, as well as the loudest ones.

If you sit quietly for 1–5 minutes twice daily, and become aware of your five senses, it brings you into the moment and helps the concentration. We are often off somewhere else in our minds, and not living in the moment.

Benefits of Relaxation

When you are relaxed, you are automatically better able to deal with everyday problems and conflicts, both at home and at work. You will find that you are not as irritable and stressed, and that your energy levels will rise. Remember too that if you are more relaxed and energised, it will have a positive effect on the people around you.

Be Spontaneous

Once you are more relaxed, another useful thing to do to enliven your life is to be spontaneous. So many of us get stuck in the routines of daily life, keeping everything under control because that is 'safe'. Letting go of control can be scary, but we can miss out on exciting opportunities in daily life because we don't see them. Try a simple change. Drop one thing that you always do, whether it's taking the same route to work every day or always doing the shopping on a certain day. Do it differently.

Making changes for the sake of change seems to excite our creativity. We are moving, making changes, seeing new things, and already life becomes more exciting. Once you allow your creativity to surface, you might find long-suppressed desires and ambitions resurfacing. Welcome these thoughts, take the time to try out some new ideas, and make time to re-kindle an old interest or hobby.

CHAPTER 8

Hormone Replacement Therapy (HRT)

What is HRT?

HRT is a chemical compound of synthetic hormones that mimic the action of the body's natural hormones, oestrogen and progesterone. HRT works by replacing the body's naturally declining levels of these hormones, i.e. during menopause, or when the ovaries are surgically removed. It has been widely promoted as a rejuvenator and a way of keeping menopause at bay.

Initially, HRT consisted of oestrogen alone. Now, oestrogen and progestogen are combined, in order to more closely mimic the body's natural activity. The idea is to trick the body into thinking that it is still pre-menopausal, in order to postpone, reduce or eliminate the symptoms of the change. The common message given out about HRT is that you will be sexier and more attractive if you take it.

Progestogens, also known as progestins or gestins, are drugs commonly now used with oestrogen as part of the HRT package. They are synthetic progesterone-analogues, such as Provera, Duphaston and Primolut. They have numerous side-effects, and possibly even cause an increase in breast cancer.

The Effects of HRT

The effects of natural and synthetic hormones on the body differ enormously. The synthetics do not match the body's chemistry, so the body is not equipped to metabolise them properly. Taking progestogen can inhibit ovulation in a menstruating woman and can produce abortion, which progesterone protects against. It can also suppress a woman's body's production of its own natural progesterone, trigger other negative side-effects and make you moody and irritable. Natural progesterone itself has none of these side-effects.

Claims that HRT protects against coronary heart disease after the menopause are spurious. Most of the evidence is conflicting. Oestrogens are believed to protect the blood vessels, and so with oestrogen levels declining at menopause, menopause brings with it greater risks of heart disease. Taking HRT, women apparently had half the risk of developing heart disease, and were less likely to die from it than the population as a whole. However, women who take HRT in general are more likely to be educated, middle-class non-smokers eating a good diet, all of which in themselves would lead to a lower risk of developing heart disease.

Is HRT Suitable for All Women?

Some women are not suitable candidates for taking HRT, that is those with a history of breast cancer in their family, or women who have had breast, ovarian or uterine cancer. Others who should avoid it are women with any type of abnormal vaginal bleeding, pancreatic disease, or who have had a recent heart attack, stroke, venous thrombosis (clots in the veins) or liver disease.

A study shows that HRT will prevent osteoporosis only if women take it for the rest of their lives, but remember that the longer it is used, the greater the risk of endometrial and breast cancer.

HRT is available in a number of different ways. It is available either as oestrogen-only, or as a combined oestrogen and progestogen preparation.

Pill Oestrogen for twenty-one or twenty-eight days a month and progestogen for between seven and twelve days each month.

Skin patch This is applied to the lower part of body and changed twice weekly.

Implant This is inserted below the skin, and lasts for six or twelve months. Progestogen must be taken orally at the same time.

Commonly Prescribed Brands of HRT

Prempak C

This form of HRT contains oestrogen and progestogen. It is used for menopausal or post-menopausal states in women who still have a uterus. It's a 'handy' form of HRT, giving an uninterrupted twenty-eight-day cycle. The progestogen counteracts cell growth — which is caused by oestrogen — in the uterus. It is prescribed for such symptoms as sweating, hot flushes, vaginitis (painful intercourse), urethritis (inflammation of the urethra) and for the prevention of osteoporosis. The dose is quite high, and there are therefore many side-effects, such as:

◆ bleeding
◆ premenstrual syndrome
◆ fibroids
◆ candida albicans
◆ cystitis
◆ cervical erosion
◆ breast tenderness
◆ nausea
◆ vomiting
◆ cramps
◆ bloating

- skin eruptions
- hair loss
- migraine
- depression
- dizziness
- weight changes
- leg cramps
- diabetes or jaundice (after prolonged use, due to an overload of steroid type).

Premarin

This contains oestrogen only. It is given to women following a hysterectomy. In the short term, it offers relief from hot flushes and other symptoms. In the long term, as part of a regime of HRT, it has been shown to reduce the risk of hip and spinal fractures in older women by as much as half, and to lower the risk of heart disease by forty to fifty per cent. However, it also has the same side effects as Prempak.

Estraderm TTS Patches

These patches are very commonly prescribed. They are available in several strengths. The patch is oestrogen only and is usually prescribed after a hysterectomy. The patch slowly releases oestrogen over a few days, therefore causing less systemic side effects, e.g. less nausea, dizziness, oedema, fibroid growth or liver disorders (because the digestive system is not involved). It is used where there are stomach ulcers, fibroids or other medication already overloading the liver. The transdermal route achieves similar oestradiol levels to those obtained with oral therapy, but at a much lower daily dose — more akin to the normal body levels of hormones pre-menopause — and also a lower oestrogen load on the liver. Adjustments to the dose can easily be made, as the oestrogen doesn't accumulate in the system to the same extent.

Estrapak 50

This contains oestrogen and progestogen, and is the lowest dose of all. It is ideal for women who are diabetic, obese or suffer other side effects of HRT. Side effects are rare, and it is always prescribed for women who still have a uterus.

Kliogest

Kliogest contains oestrogen and progestogen in high doses. It is mainly indicated for treatment of oestrogen deficiency syndromes and prevention of bone mineral content loss in post menopausal women, especially where there is a family history of, or diagnosis of, osteoporosis. It can cause atrophy of the uterus. It is not recommended for use in women with a family history of breast or uterine cancer, or thrombosis or hypertension.

Oestrogel

Oestrogel is oestrogen only in gel form, applied to arms, shoulders or inner thighs, never the breasts or vulval region. It has few systemic side effects, but as the absorption rates are high — it enters the blood stream directly, and is not subject to the digestive process — there is very little dose control. It is not recommended for patients with fibroids or a family history of uterine cancer. It may cause fluid retention, leading to hypertension and cardiac dysfunction. It bypasses the portal system, so is therefore easier on the liver; it is therefore suitable for those on other medication.

How Safe is HRT?

The answer is that no one really knows. HRT hasn't been around for long enough yet in order to fully evaluate its effects on health — it has only been prescribed in the last twenty to twenty-five years.

Risks of HRT

Endometrial cancer There is a risk of endometrial cancer with the use of HRT. This happened in the 1960s and 1970s, when only oestrogen was used. Sixty out of one hundred women developed endometrial malignancies within five years of treatment. Adding progesterone to the treatment lowered the risk of contracting endometrial cancer over oestrogen-alone preparations, but the combined drug still increases your endometrial cancer risk by up to one-third over those who don't take HRT.

Ovarian cancer There is said to be a small increase in the risk of developing ovarian cancer, but no concrete proof.

Breast cancer There are conflicting results concerning whether there is an increased risk of breast cancer for women who are on HRT. It is worse if there is a family history of breast cancer. At least three major studies show that the risk of breast cancer doubles with the use of HRT after six years. A Swedish study also shows that, far from protecting against breast cancer, the addition of progestogen actually quadruples the risk after four years.

Blood pressure Blood pressure is likely to rise, although this is only at the commencement of treatment.

Weight gain This also happens only at the start of treatment.

Bleeding Periods will usually continue between eighty and ninety per cent while a woman is on HRT. You will have some shorter and lighter periods, and at other times have severe bleeding.

Any strong, orthodox medicine is going to have side effects. We were not aware of the effects of steroids until some time after they were introduced. At this stage, we just don't know what the long-term side effects will be of HRT. Also, when you stop taking HRT you tend to have menopausal symptoms, so in fact taking HRT will only postpone menopause.

Menopausal women are not ill — you may never get any of the illnesses that HRT is supposed to prevent. Your symptoms can be dealt with by non-drug means, so why are women given a drug that has the side effect of causing life-threatening disease?

CHAPTER 9

Homeopathy — How It Can Help During Menopause

What is Homeopathy?

Homeopathy is a complete system of medicine, which aims to promote general health by reinforcing the body's own natural healing capacity. It does not treat physical, emotional, mental or even spiritual illnesses separately, but regards them all as being interconnected, since they are all part of the patient's suffering.

Homeopaths recognise that each person is an individual; as each individual reacts to their illnesses in their own unique way, so the homeopath will prescribe a remedy, not merely for their symptoms but for their whole state. Homeopathy works in quite a different way to conventional medicine. Conventional medicine takes the view that symptoms are a direct manifestation of the illness. So, drugs are given which work against the disease and its symptoms. Therefore we have antibiotics, anti-depressants, anti-inflammatories, etc., treating only the local illness and not the underlying cause.

The word homeopathy comes from two Greek words meaning 'similar' and 'suffering', the practice of treating like with like. That is to say, treating an illness with a substance that produces similar symptoms to those displayed by the person who is ill. Homeopaths call this the Law of Similars. This law states 'That which makes sick shall heal'. This means that the symptoms caused by an overdose of a substance are the symptoms that can also be cured with a small dose of that substance. For example, we know that when cutting an onion, we often experience stinging, runny eyes, and a burning, runny nose. These symptoms are typical of hay fever, so hay fever sufferers with these symptoms will be helped by the remedy made from onion, *Allium cepa*.

The Law of Similars was known to Hippocrates, the fifth-century Greek physician, and to the Swiss alchemist Paracelsus in the sixteenth century, both of whom recognised the role of nature as the curer of diseases.

Are Homeopathic Remedies Safe?

Homeopathic remedies are safe and non-addictive. This is because only very minute amounts of the active ingredients are used in the preparation. The remedies come from many different sources. Most are derived from plants, but metals, minerals and some poisons which have been used medicinally for generations are also used. The remedies are made by serial dilution and succussion (vigorous shaking either by hand or by machine) in a solution of alcohol and water. This is repeated many times, from a few up to many thousand times.

The liquid dilution can then be used as a remedy itself, or used to medicate tablets or granules. The remedies are called 'potentised' and, depending on the number of dilutions and succussions they have undertaken, are given numbers, i.e. 6c, 12c, 30c, 200c, 1m, etc. The higher the number, the more the remedy has been diluted and succussed, and the stronger it becomes. It is more powerful and longer acting than the lower strengths, and is usually only prescribed by experienced, qualified homeopaths.

Our Own Natural Healing Powers

We all have natural healing powers within us to cope with the stresses and strains of everyday life. When we are 'healthy' we recover very quickly. But a point may be reached where the external stresses on any level become so great that in order to defend, repair and maintain order in the system, the healing powers have to produce symptoms and signs of what we call an illness, or disease. If our vitality is low, then our susceptibility to illness will be high.

What is the Purpose of Symptoms?

The healing powers are continually trying to maintain order in the system, but once the external stresses reach a certain level, this can't be done passively and the attempt to keep a balance produces outward signs which we generally find uncomfortable. If we look at it in this way, the symptoms and signs of disease appear different. They are no longer the inconvenient, un-wanted, useless and 'why did I have to get it now' things they are commonly thought to be, but they are actually the manifesta-tion of each person's attempt to get well, to maintain order and balance in the system. *They are the external effects of the internal fight to get well, recover and heal. They are not a part of becoming ill, but are a part of the healing process.*

Now it becomes clearer why, in a young healthy child where 'disease' serves its function in its most simple and natural form, it has been observed that the child is 'better' after an acute illness than before it. It is also understandable why people tend to become 'ill' when there are a lot of stresses going on in their lives, and especially at times of crises such as grief, changes in work and marriage break-ups. Quite simply, these are times when there is more healing to be done, when more effort is required by the natural healing powers to maintain order, and it is no longer possible for a balance to be sustained without the production of symptoms of disease. In the same way, if a woman finds the menopause a stressful time, she will produce symptoms such as menstrual irregularities, hot flushes, irritability, etc.

How Does Homeopathy Fit into this Picture of Disease?

Once it is understood that the symptoms of disease are actually a good thing, in that they are the outward indication of the healing and balancing process that is going on inside each individual person, then to give a medicine that is capable of mimicking and bringing about that same process seems to be a good idea. It's logical.

Homeopathy and Menopause

Homeopathy is a truly holistic medicine. This means that we observe the person on all levels and regard the spiritual, mental, emotional and physical aspects of the person to be completely interconnected. If a woman consults a homeopath with menopausal problems — say hot flushes only — the homeopath will still look at the person as a whole, and not just prescribe a remedy for the hot flushes. This is called a constitutional remedy.

If we prescribe in this way, the overall imbalance will be treated, the person's hot flushes will go and their overall health will be improved. Sometimes, we come across people who have no other problems in their life, who just present with some specific menopausal symptoms; in these cases, prescribing on those symptoms alone will solve the problem.

It is preferable to be treated by an experienced homeopath, but there are some remedies that you could try yourself. I have given details below of some of the more common homeopathic remedies prescribed during the menopause. I have suggested the 30c potency as a good potency to use. If you follow the directions below for recommended dosages and repetitions, you will do yourself no harm.

Directions for Taking Homeopathic Remedies

Do not eat or drink for fifteen minutes before and after taking the remedy. You should avoid coffee, camphor, menthol, peppermint, eucalyptus and other strong-smelling substances during the course of treatment, as these can interfere with your remedy. Dissolve the remedy on the tongue, one tablet daily for three days, then wait for an improvement. If there is no change after three to four weeks, select a more appropriate remedy. If there is improvement, wait until there is a return of the symptoms, then repeat the dose.

It is important that the remedy, once it has worked, is allowed to complete its action. Do not repeat the remedy too soon. Wait for the return of symptoms. This is often the most difficult thing for people to do! If there is no improvement in your symptoms, consult your homeopath, or your doctor.

I have listed below some of the homeopathic remedies which are most often needed during menopause.

Lachesis

Lachesis is an important remedy during the menopause, and is often called for in women who have never felt well since the onset of menopause. Other menopausal symptoms of this remedy are:

◆ haemorrhages
◆ fainting
◆ weakness
◆ melancholy
◆ periods every twenty-one days
◆ periods profuse

- generally worse before menses, and pains and mood better once the flow starts
- hot flushes, with headaches, palpitations and hot sweats
- headaches, especially in the vertex, with burning sensations
- some nausea, diarrhoea or haemorrhoids.

The left ovary can also be painful and swollen, and there may also be prolapsed uterus. Women may be asthmatic since reaching the menopause. They generally feel worse in the mornings, can't stand the heat and are hypersensitive to any tight clothing at the neck or waist.

The remedy is prepared from the venom of *Lachesis muta*, the surucuccu snake of South America.

Recommended dosage: One dose daily for three days of *Lachesis* 30c, to be taken as directed above.

Sepia

Sepia is mainly a female remedy. It is known as the 'washerwoman's remedy', because people who need this remedy:

- are worn down
- exhausted
- weepy
- weak
- perspire profusely
- need air
- must sit down and cross their legs, as they feel their insides will fall out
- are so worn out they can appear indifferent to their loved ones.

They have a sharp tongue, and almost take pleasure from hurting loved ones. This is not because they don't love their family, it's because they are just worn out and exhausted and have nothing more to give to anyone. A woman who was formerly warm and loving is now saying 'I don't have any emotions'; sometimes she will say she can't even remember the sensation or feeling of happiness or joy. She can feel she must hold on to something to prevent herself from screaming. She can have dullness of mind, feel stupid and absent-minded, with no initiative.

Physically, during the menopause she may have a dry vagina, pain on intercourse, lack of desire or aversion to sex. She may have flooding during periods, sudden flushes of heat, weakness, perspiration and a sinking feeling in the pit of her stomach. In general, she feels better from activity, especially in the open air, and better from warmth and from eating. She also feels better after sleep, even a short nap (this is the opposite of *Lachesis*). She generally feels worse in the evenings.

Sepia is a very useful remedy at the menopause. It is prepared from the liquid found in the ink sac of the cuttlefish, *Sepia officinalis*. The shape of the cuttlefish is reminiscent of the uterus. The sex organs of the cuttlefish are right down at the end.

The remedy *Sulphuric acid* is sometimes needed to complete the action of *Sepia*.

Recommended dosage: One dose daily for three days of Sepia 30c, to be taken as directed above.

Sulphuric Acid

This is another very useful remedy during menopause. Like all the acids, weakness and debility are common to this remedy, especially in the digestive tract, giving a very relaxed feeling to the stomach, and a craving for stimulants. They feel a weakness out of all proportion to the problem. It affects the blood and blood vessels, causing haemorrhages of thin, black blood.

Other symptoms of this remedy are:

◆ prolapse of vagina and uterus from weakness
◆ flushes of heat, followed by sweating and a trembling all over
◆ irritability
◆ weepiness over the slightest thing.

They can have nightmares before or after periods. They must do everything in a hurry. They get angry and impatient because things move so slowly. No one does anything to please them.

This remedy is made from sulphuric acid.

Recommended dosage: One dose daily for three days of Sulphuric acid 30c, to be taken as directed above.

Folliculinum

From extensive research done by the American homeopath, Melissa Assilem, she has seen that many women had symptoms between ovulation and menses and many of them had taken the Pill in the past, or their mothers had taken the Pill before they were conceived. This is a very useful remedy for women with hormonal symptoms who may have used the Pill, and also useful for symptoms during the menopause.

Melissa Assilem says: 'Folliculinum is a really brilliant remedy around menopause. It pretty well covers the whole range of physical and mental symptoms we might find at this time.'

There will often be a history of abuse, sexual, physical or psychological. The woman may have had a very strict up-bringing. She can be unfocused, feel 'spaced' and may totally lose herself in her relationships.

Assilem expands on the symptoms: 'She becomes addicted to rescuing people. She feels drained. She has become a door-mat. She has forgotten who she is. She has no individuality.'

Folliculinum can help restore the will and re-empower the person. It is generally seen after this remedy that the person takes control of her life again, finds her own identity, becomes her own rescuer and won't allow herself to be used ever again. It allows people to break the patterns from the past that they find hard to change. It helps to restore clarity.

Possible physical symptoms of *Folliculinum* during menopause:

- restless, hyperactive, worse at rest
- dizziness and faintness
- puts on weight without overeating, as much as 7 lb/3 kg before menses
- huge food cravings, especially for sugar, sweets
- cycle irregularities
- flooding
- hot flushes, night sweats
- abdominal heaviness
- fibroids
- vaginal dryness.

This remedy is made from oestrone, a synthetic form of oestrogen.

Recommended dosage: One dose daily for three days of *Folliculinum* 30c, to be taken as directed above.

Calcium Carbonicum

Calcium carbonicum (*Calc. carb.*) is a very useful remedy during the menopause. The typical *Calc. carb.* woman is responsible, dutiful and hard-working, 'a pillar of the community'. She can take on too many responsibilities and become overwhelmed by them. Mentally, she can be tired and unable to hold on to thoughts or details, and then she feels that she is going mad and worries that other people will realise it. She has always worried about what others think of her and even more so now. She has a strong focus on security, with lots of anxieties around money and health. When she is ill, she can despair of ever recovering her health.

You can imagine a *Calc. carb.* woman if she develops troublesome symptoms during the menopause. She will worry about her health, she can think she will never feel 'normal' again. She will worry about her family, her children and her husband should anything happen to her. She will be anxious about the future.

Some physical menopausal symptoms experienced by women who need *Calc. carb.* are:

◆ hot flushes, with burning sensations in the vertex
◆ head and neck wet with perspiration, worse during sleep
◆ metrorrhagia and uterine fibroids, sometimes with marked uterine haemorrhages.

This remedy is prepared from the middle layer of the oyster shell. The soft, white, calcareous substance is secreted by the mantle of the mollusc, and is a deposit of finely crystalline calcium carbonate.

Recommended dosage: One dose daily for three days of *Calc. carb.* 30c, to be taken as directed above.

Cimicifuga Racemosa

The *Cimicifuga* patient can be very loquacious (like *Lachesis*), jumping from one subject to another quickly. They are excitable, extroverted and forceful. Emotionally, they can be hysterical at times. They have strong phobias, such as insanity and death. They are restless and can appear frantic. Their moods can be changeable and they can be gloomy and morose. They can be depressed and describe it as if a black cloud were sitting on top of them.

One of the keynotes of *Cimicifuga* is alternation of physical and mental symptoms. So, mental symptoms improve when physical symptoms are present. They tend to feel worse during menses, worse for the flow (opposite of *Lachesis*).

Typical physical symptoms are:

- irregular periods, which may be suppressed by emotions or stress
- neuralgic pains in the ovaries
- bearing down pains, suggesting uterine prolapse, along with pains across pelvis and shooting down the thighs
- extreme tenderness of ovaries and uterus
- left-sided symptoms predominate (*Lachesis*)
- hot flushes with a pale, ashen face and a cold forehead
- general aggravation from cold, and relief from warmth in every form.

This remedy is also known as *Actaea racemosa*, or black cohosh. It is a member of the *Ranunculaceae* family, a perennial herb, found in deep woods in eastern North America. The plant was used medicinally by North American Indian women for rheumatism, menstrual disorders, slow parturition and snakebite.

Recommended dosage: One dose daily for three days of *Cimicifuga* 30c, to be taken as directed above.

Pulsatilla

Pulsatilla is a very important remedy for women's complaints and is often of use during the menopause. The woman needing this remedy is of a gentle, mild disposition. She is emotional and easily moved to laughter or tears. Her moods are changeable; she can cry at every little thing and loves to be comforted. She can also be easily irritated and has a tendency to feel slighted, or be fearful of being slighted. In general, she feels better in the fresh air and feels worse in a warm, stuffy room and in the evenings.

Physical problems include irregular menstruation, whether it is too early or too late, too scanty or too profuse. The menses can be painful enough to cause nausea or vomiting, and the pains can be helped by bending double. Unusually, the bleeding can happen during the day only. She can have difficulty sleeping because of hot flushes and anxious thoughts, and her legs can be very restless at night.

The remedy is prepared from *Pulsatilla nigricans*, the wind-flower, meadow anemone, or pasque flower, and is a member of the Ranunculaceae family. It is native to Scandinavia, Denmark, Germany and Russia. The whole fresh-flowering plant is used in the preparation of the remedy.

Recommended dosage: One dose daily for three days of *Pulsatilla* 30c, to be taken as directed above.

CHAPTER 10

Case Histories

The cases in this chapter are factual, but I have changed the patients' names.

I hope you will see from these cases the importance of always looking for a remedy for the whole person, not just for the menopausal symptoms. Not every woman with hot flushes during the menopause will need *Lachesis*, and yet it is the first remedy that will come to mind. It is essential always to look at the patient as a whole, to discover the overall imbalance and see what she is finding most difficult to cope with at this time. Is it the hot flushes or other physical symptoms? Is she finding the emotional ups and downs, the irritability and the panic attacks most difficult? Look for anything unusual — for anything that will differentiate this person from the next one. Find a remedy to match the whole picture, and the woman will feel better and there will be an improvement in her symptoms.

Case One
Joan

Joan, aged forty-eight, came to see me in July 1994, complaining of hot flushes during the day and profuse perspiration at night in bed. The latter was causing her a lot of stress, as it was interrupting her sleep; she had to change her clothes about three times every night. Joan said that she was very moody, irritable, tense and weepy. She generally felt worse when she woke up in the mornings. She was also very low in energy. At that time, Joan had had no periods for six months, and they were light and irregular before that. Joan is a very witty person, who loves to talk.

Treatment

I prescribed one dose of *Lachesis* 200c.

Short-Term Outcome

When Joan returned a month later, the hot flushes had diminished by about ninety per cent. She said that her moods were more stable, and she was in great form. She had a light period, which lasted for a few days, during the month. Her energy had come back up, and she was happier in herself.

Long-Term Outcome

Over the next few months, her hot flushes went completely, and she had another light period. Her mood and energy continued to be good. Six months later, with the slight return of her symptoms, I repeated the *Lachesis* 200c and Joan has been symptom-free now for about two years.

Case Two
Marie

Forty-nine-year-old Marie came to see me in November 1995, with headaches, usually during the week before her periods, mainly over the left eye. She described the pain as shooting outwards, and it was made worse by lying on the affected side. Her hair was falling out. She was getting sudden flushes of heat, with weakness and sweating. Marie had weak, dragging, bearing down pains — she felt as if everything would escape from her vulva. She also had breakthrough bleeding. She was tired all the time. 'I'm worn out,' she said. Everything piles up at home — the washing, ironing, beds to be made, etc. Marie was worse in the evenings, feeling exhausted at that time of the day. She had no interest in sex, as she was simply too tired.

Treatment
I prescribed one dose of *Sepia*, 200c.

Short-Term Outcome
After four to six weeks, Marie returned with a smile on her face. She had much more energy, her headaches were gone, and the flushes of heat much reduced. The dragging pains she felt were not as bad as they had been, and there was some improvement in the breakthrough bleeding. It would probably take a few months for that to regulate. She said 'I am back to my old self.' She had more interest in her husband, and her mood and humour were much improved.

Long-Term Outcome
The headaches never returned and the flushes of heat gradually diminished. The breakthrough bleeding stopped after a few months. She came to see me about ten months later with some slight return of symptoms. She was feeling tired, had had some hot flushes and felt some dragging down pains. Her son was causing some anxiety — he had got into trouble, and Marie was feeling stressed by it all. I felt that this had stopped the action of the remedy, and repeated *Sepia* 200c. Marie was back to her old self soon afterwards, and felt more able to cope with her son's problems.

Case Three
Margaret

Margaret, aged fifty-one, came to see me in January 1996, complaining of having had hot flushes for a couple of months. She felt hot from the neck upwards, and was perspiring a lot on her head and neck. Her legs were restless at night. She had recently become constipated. Margaret's periods had been irregular for some time, and she had had none for nine months. She said she had become short-tempered with her husband and the children. She was worried about her health and about the future. She has four children.

Margaret has worked hard all her life looking after her four children, and has never had time for herself. At the time of her first visit to me, her youngest child had reached the age of eighteen, and she was wondering what she would do now that her children would not need her as much. She is a very dependable person. She has always worried about what other people think of her. In terms of food, she has strong desires for eggs, salt and sweet things.

Treatment

I prescribed one dose of *Calcium carbonate*, 200c.

Short-Term Outcome

After six weeks, Margaret returned. 'The hot flushes are gone,' she said. Her legs were not as restless at night. She had more energy, and had decided to do a course in creative writing. She used to like writing as a teenager, but when the children came along she didn't have the time. Maybe she'll write a bestseller one of these days!

Long-Term Outcome

Margaret needed to repeat *Calcium carbonate*, 200c, about three months later, and for the past year she has had no problems.

Case Four
Elizabeth

Forty-nine-year-old Elizabeth came to see me in December 1996. 'I'm going through the menopause,' she said. She was tired, cranky, tearful. Her father had died six months previously. She had looked after her father since her mother died two years ago. She never married — any relationships she has had in the past all ended disastrously. She felt angry about a lot of things that happened in the past, but was afraid of her anger and couldn't express it.

When she visited me, Elizabeth was in a relationship with a man who was separated from his wife. She felt angry and tearful. Her partner blamed her for everything that went wrong. 'How dare he!' she said, but was afraid to say that to him. At that time, Elizabeth felt that she was at a crossroads in her life. Her moods were changeable, and her periods very irregular.

Treatment

I prescribed *Staphisagria*, LM1, one dose daily.

Short-Term Outcome

Elizabeth returned five weeks later. She said that she had cried a lot during that time; she also had a heavy cold for a week. Her moods were much better and she had a period after thirty days. She made some changes in her life too, including splitting up with the separated man. She was very assertive at work, and overall she felt that she was taking control of her life for the first time.

Long-Term Outcome

Over the next six months or so, Elizabeth continued on *Staphisagria*, going from LM1 to LM4. During that time she met an interesting man, and was hoping that this relationship would work out. She was no longer afraid to express how she feels and became much more assertive as a person.

Case Five
Helen

Helen, aged forty-eight, came to see me in August 1995. She complained of hot flushes; poor concentration; headaches (which she described as dull, all consuming, that could last for days); tiredness that was worse in the early afternoons; and sleep difficulties, with hot sweats waking her every two hours. When she was about forty, she had very heavy, painful periods, and was diagnosed with fibroids and cysts on her ovaries. She had a hysterectomy. A few years later, Helen was put on HRT because of her mood swings. Some two years later, she developed lumps in her breasts — which were removed — and she then went off HRT.

Helen is happily married, with two children. She is an independent person, and can be stubborn if she thinks she is in the right. She wouldn't want to be a burden to anyone. She is a sensitive person. She likes the house to be neat and tidy, but is not obsessive. She does administrative work in an office and likes things to be orderly. If criticised, she withdraws into herself. She is very sensitive to cruelty to others. She frequently gets upset while watching the television. She fears spiders and heights. At the time of her first visit to me, Helen had had lots of chest infections and was suffering from constipation. She loves fish, eggs and vegetables.

Treatment

I prescribed *Calcium carbonate*, LM1, one dose daily.

Short-Term Outcome

Helen returned five weeks later for a consultation. She said 'Things don't affect me as much. I'm more level, more calm than I was.' She was sleeping better, not waking up with hot flushes. She had had no headaches at all since the initial visit, and her constipation went.

Long-Term Outcome

She continued on the remedy for a few months, going from
LM1 to LM4 when some hot flushes returned in the day
and a few at night. Helen then went off the remedy, the hot
flushes disappeared, and she has been symptom-free for the
last year.

Case Six
Sue

Sue came to see me in August 1996 at the age of forty-eight,
suffering from exhaustion. She has three teenagers and a
cranky, domineering husband who expects high standards of
everyone. She has a full-time job in the local factory. Her
sister's son had recently come to work in Dublin and was
living with the family.

Physically, Sue was exhausted, had dizzy spells and felt
faint in the heat. She was drained, and felt weak. She was
suffering from hot flushes, a swollen abdomen, had sugar cravings and the migraines she had had for years were worse than
ever. 'Superwoman'! No wonder Sue was exhausted.

Even with all these symptoms, Sue was still getting on
with her job and looking after everyone. She is the 'rescuer'
of the family, helping everyone else, with no time for herself.
She has a history of being on the Pill for about eight years,
prescribed for premenstrual tension, heavy periods and
swollen breasts before menses. She also has a history of
candida albicans.

Treatment

I prescribed *Folliculinum*, 30c, once daily for three days.

Short-Term Outcome

Sue's symptoms cleared up, the migraines went and she was
much stronger and brighter in herself. Her desire for sugar

reduced considerably and her energy level went up. She continued working in her job, but no longer allowed her children or her husband to weigh her down with their demands. She started line dancing and even went away for a couple of dancing weekends, leaving her family to look after themselves. She finally started to have some fun in her life!

Long-Term Outcome

Sue came back to see me five months later — she had relapsed slightly. I repeated *Folliculinum*, 30c, and repeated the remedy again six months later. She continues to be well.

Case Seven
Ann

Ann, aged forty-seven, came to see me with period problems. She had dark, stringy clots of blood and she talked about the sensation of something moving about in her abdomen. She had hot flushes, and complained of a sensation of crawling under the skin at the same time, which she was finding very distressing. She also had tingling noises in her ears. Emotionally, Ann was moody, swinging from highs to lows. She got cross with her husband over silly things, and immediately felt very sorry, but she was not able to help it. She said that she had a short fuse. These were the main symptoms of the case.

Treatment

One dose of the remedy *Crocus* 200c helped her enormously.

Short-Term Outcome

Ann returned to see me six weeks later. Her periods were not as stringy — there was more of a flow. Her ears had cleared completely — 'such a relief' she said. She was still getting cross at times with her husband, but didn't immediately feel sorry! The hot flushes were much improved, not happening as often as before. She felt there was a gentle improvement overall.

Long-Term Outcome

I repeated the remedy three months later, and Ann continues to improve all the time.

To finish, I would like to share a poem with you which I think says it all about women's experiences during the menopause. I hope you enjoy it and that you find it inspiring.

These women
These others
Who have lost the blossom of youth.
These women who have laugh lines and looser skin
And the deepest eyes
Where you swim in compassion, wisdom and truth.
These women of fifty
Who laugh easily and can hold the whole world in their
    hearts.
They've grieved the loss of youth,
They've grown through the children leaving home,
They've seen partners age
And go away.
They've seen death.
From where do they get their bloom?
From where do they blush of yet unknown pleasures?
For blush they do.
Discovery and delight are still in their repertoire.
They know themselves
And they know life.
Their laugh is a giggle of groundedness.
They've experienced so much.
Their power grows.
Their creative force is no longer present in pert breasts,
Rather the well-hung fullness of ripened fruit.
The world needs them, for they carry the sweetness and
    mysteries of life.
They carry the questions.
They carry the answers.
Their souls run deep.

They fashion wisdom from the experiences of days gone
  by.
They are alive with lustiness for life.
The lustiness that comes from knowing
They are beautiful.
Well-worn, comfortable, easy
Like your favourite chair.
No fragile beauty here.
They're solid, with the delicious delicacy that comes with
  age.
These women.
These women of fifty
Who lust for love, laughter, and life,
Who live long and hard and deep.
These women who wrestle with life.
These women who dare to know their spirits.
Their hearts glow.
Their bodies quiver.
They are on the brink.
A man is lucky to know one,
To have one in his life.
These women are treasures.
Gems.
They will set you ablaze if you care to come in close.
These women of fifty are fire and earth
And their breath can take you away
Or give you life.
Their knowing goes deeper than you can even imagine
Yet their vision is clear and supple and flexible.
These women
These women of fifty.

Helene Kass, Columbia, Maryland, USA

Charts

1. DIETARY CHART	
INCREASE	**DECREASE**
Quality of food you eat.	*Quantity* Reduce the quantity of food you consume. Eat less but eat nutritious food.
Unrefined, unprocessed and organic food. Put as little stress on the body as possible by eating food that has been tampered with as little as possible, i.e. unrefined, unprocessed and organic food.	*Refined*, processed food. Eat less refined, processed or 'convenience' foods, which if eaten consistently can put a stress on the body.
Fibre Eat more foods high in fibre, i.e. wholemeal flour, bread, potatoes, pasta, brown rice, peas, beans, lentils, vegetables, dried fruit and unsalted nuts.	*Sugar* Lower your sugar intake. It is addictive and will cause mood swings of highs and lows. Be careful of sugar in cakes, biscuits, tinned fruit, fizzy drinks, jams and sweet breakfast cereals. Look for hidden sugars, e.g. in baked beans. *continued*

1. DIETARY CHART contd

INCREASE contd	DECREASE contd
Fats, Oils and Spreads When using oils and spreads, use more Olive oil, Sunflower oil, non-hydrogenated oils and spreads, low-fat cheeses, skimmed or semi-skimmed milk.	*Fats* Lower your fat intake — especially from animal sources, red meat, crisps, chocolate, cakes, biscuits, full-fat cheeses, saturated oils and spreads, full-cream milk, cream, butter and ice cream.
Seasoning Use lemon, herbs, spices and mustard for seasoning, instead of salt. Sea salt is preferable to table salt because it contains valuable minerals especially iodine but keep it to a minimum.	*Salt* Reduce salt. Watch out for salty snacks, crisps and salted nuts. Make homemade soups, as packets and tinned soups have hidden salt. Look for 'no added salt' on labels.
Fluids Increase your water intake, drink at least 4 pints of water daily. Old Naturopaths suggest 8 pints daily!	*Fluids* Cut down on the quantity of tea, coffee and alcohol you drink.

2. GENERAL HORMONAL CHART

INCREASE	DECREASE
Carrots, ripe bananas, apples, celery, broccoli, leafy greens, cucumber, all berries, papaya, seeds/sprouted, linseed, soya flour, soya products, walnuts, avocado, kelp, liquorice and alfalfa.	Caffeine, dairy products, fats, fries, junk food, red meat, sugar and fizzy drinks.

Helpful Extras
Evening Primrose oil, Agnus Castus, Rescue Remedy, Royal Jelly, Geranium Essential Oil (good hormone balancer), or Female Essence by Jan de Vries.

3. VITAMINS & MINERALS CHART

INCREASE	DECREASE
Hormone Balance Calcium, Vitamin D, Magnesium, Phosphorus, Vitamin K, Manganese, Zinc, Vitamin B Complex, Vitamin C and Boron.	
Calcium To hold on to calcium in the body include the following substances in your diet: seaweed, dairy products, canned fish, nuts, seeds especially sesame, soya products, tofu, spinach, cabbage, broccoli, beans, figs, apricots, black treacle, wholegrains, pulses.	*Calcium* To prevent the loss of calcium from the body, reduce the following foods in your diet: red meat, all protein, salt, coffee, rhubarb, spinach, brown rice, sugar and a high-fat diet.
Calcium Supplements Floradix Calcium *or* Bioforce Urticalcin *or* Nature's Own Foodstate Calcium *or* Vitabiotics Osteocare *or* Lifeplan Sea Kelp.	

continued

3. VITAMINS & MINERALS CHART contd

INCREASE *contd*	DECREASE *contd*
Calcium is more effective when taken in smaller doses throughout the day; when taken at night it promotes a sound sleep.	
Magnesium	*Magnesium*
Magnesium is vital to enzyme activity and assists the body in calcium and potassium uptake. It is found in such foods as dairy products, fish, meat and seafood. Other foods rich in magnesium are green leafy vegetables, sesame seeds, soya beans, nuts, cashews, almonds, brazils, peanuts, brewer's yeast, brown rice, figs, apples, avocados, bananas, apricots, lemons, grapefruit, yellow corn, garlic, wheat and whole grains.	Decrease your intake of alcohol, as this increases your body's need for magnesium. Foods that inhibit the absorption of magnesium include large amounts of fats, cod liver oil, calcium, Vitamin D and protein.
Magnesium Supplements	
Sona Magnesium *or* Sona CalMag *or* Magnesium OK.	
	continued

3. VITAMINS & MINERALS CHART contd	
INCREASE contd	*DECREASE contd*
Boron Boron is needed in trace amounts for calcium absorption and for healthy bones. A study in America indicated that, within eight days of menopausal women supplementing their diet with 3 mg of boron, they lost 40% less calcium, one-third less magnesium, and slightly less phosphorus through their urine. (Do not take more than 3 mg daily.) Boron is found in such foods as leafy vegetables, dairy products, fish, meat, soya beans, prunes, raisins, nuts, grains and honey. *Boron Supplements* Boron Tablets *or* Confiance *or* Menopace.	

4. HOT FLUSHES/SWEATS CHART

INCREASE	*DECREASE*
Sage tea or tincture can be taken as an infusion. Liquidise cucumbers and add to a pint of water — take a glass before bedtime. Bananas and Oranges. Regular deep breathing helps, as does relaxation. Take regular physical exercise, turn your central heating down and keep your rooms well ventilated.	Alcohol, *stress* and anxiety, hot drinks, caffeine, cigarettes, spicy food, sugar, additives and hot baths.

Supplements
Vitamin C, Vitamin E (very important), Siberian Ginseng, Potassium, Evening Primrose Oil, Bioforce Menosan.

Homeopathic Remedies
Lachesis, Graphites, Pulsatilla, Sulphuric Acid or Amylenum Nitrosum.

5. ANXIETY/DEPRESSION CHART

INCREASE	DECREASE
Zinc, found in oysters, herrings, milk, meat, eggs, cheese, whole grains, cereals, pulses and seeds. Deep breathing, exercise, yoga and meditation. Rosemary, basil and hops in cooking or herbal teas. *Supplements or Oils* Vitamin B Complex, Zinc, St John's Wort (Hypericum), Bioforce Ginsavita and Valerian. Neroli Essential Oil, Lavender Oil or Chamomile Essential Oil could be used in the bath, in a burner or mixed with base oil for massage.	*Caffeine* in such substances as coffee, tea, cola and chocolate.

6. IRREGULAR PERIODS CHART

INCREASE	DECREASE
Iron, in such foods as eggs, fish, liver, meat, poultry, green leafy vegetables, whole grains, and enriched breads and cereals. Other food sources include almonds, avocados, beets, blackstrap molasses, brewer's yeast, dates, figs, dulse, egg yolks, kelp, kidney and lima beans, lentils, millet, parsley, peaches, pears, dried prunes, pumpkins, raisins, rice and wheat bran, sesame seeds and soybeans.	
Vitamin C with iron can increase iron absorption as much as 30%. Sources of Vitamin C are green vegetables, berries and citrus fruits. It is found in asparagus, avocados, beet greens, broccoli, Brussels sprouts, cantaloupe melon, currants, grapefruit, kale, lemons, mangoes, mustard greens, onions, oranges, papayas, parsley, green peas, sweet peppers, persimmons,	*continued*

6. IRREGULAR PERIODS CHART contd

INCREASE contd	DECREASE contd
pineapple, radishes, rose hips, spinach, strawberries, Swiss chard, tomatoes, turnip greens and watercress. *Zinc*, found in fish, vegetables, meats, oysters, poultry, seafood and whole grains. Also brewer's yeast, egg yolks, lamb chops, liver, mushrooms, pecan nuts, pumpkin seeds, sardines, seeds, soya lecithin, soya beans and sunflower seeds. *Supplements* Floradix or Spatone (Iron), Vitamin C, Vitamin B Complex, Zinc, Evening Primrose Oil.	

7. DRYNESS/GENITAL CHANGES & LOSS OF LIBIDO CHART

INCREASE	DECREASE
Vitamin E is found in the following foods: cold-pressed vegetable oils, whole grains, dark-green leafy vegetables, nuts and seeds, eggs, organ meats, wheat germ, oatmeal and milk. *Extract of wild Mexican yam*, in substances such as Natragest, ProGest, Progone Cream (Irish) or Perfect Woman herbal vaginal cream.	

8. ANGER/IRRITABILITY CHART

INCREASE	DECREASE
Chamomile Essential Oil is very calming. It can be used in the bath, in a burner or mixed with a base oil for massage.	Stimulants such as coffee, tea, cola.

9. FREQUENCY OF URINATION & INCONTINENCE CHART

INCREASE	DECREASE
Vitamin E. Extract of wild Mexican yam in the form of creams. Increase your water intake to at least 4 pints daily. Wearing loose cotton underwear will help prevent irritation of the urogential tract. Pelvic floor exercises.	

10. POOR MEMORY & CONCENTRATION CHART

INCREASE	DECREASE
Oily fish, such as mackerel, herrings and sardines. Dark green and orange vegetables, liver, nuts and shellfish. Use the herb Rosemary in cooking. It is the best memory enhancer. Keep the brain active — study something you're interested in. Your brain is like a muscle. The more you use it the better it becomes. *Supplements* Iron, Betacarotene, Gingko Biloba, Coenzyme Q-10, Multi B Vitamin with Vitamins B1 and B12, Choline, Zinc, Magnesium and Calcium.	

11. INSOMNIA CHART

INCREASE	DECREASE
St John's Wort (Hypericum), warm milk, take a long walk or some aerobic exercise an hour before bed.	

12. OSTEOPOROSIS CHART

INCREASE

Take more exercise. Weight-bearing exercises maintain strong healthy bones and protect you against osteoporosis. If unfit, introduce exercise gently in the form of walking, swimming, yoga, t'ai chi, dancing or gardening.

Increase your intake of Calcium, Magnesium and Boron.

Take two essential fatty acids — GLA (gamma linolenic acid) which is in Evening Primrose Oil and EPA (eicosapentaenoic acid) which is found in fish oils.

The use of natural plant-derived progesterone in such creams as Natragest, Pro-Gest, Progone and Perfect Woman.

DECREASE

Try to get rid of the stress in your life. Stop smoking: studies have shown that stopping smoking reduced the risk of osteoporotic fractures. Reduce your intake of highly processed, over-refined foods, high-fat foods, red meats, all protein, salt, coffee and alcohol. Throw out your aluminium saucepans!

13. PANIC ATTACK CHART

INCREASE	DECREASE
Deep breathing is invaluable in cases of panic attacks. The Bach Flower remedy 'Rock Rose' can also help.	

Useful Addresses

Irish Society of Homeopaths
Ruxton Court, 35 Dominick Street, Galway. Tel. 091 565040.

The Irish Society of Homeopaths is the professional body for practising Classical Homeopaths in Ireland. It publishes a register listing qualified and experienced homeopaths who have agreed to abide by the Society's code of ethics. These homeopaths are issued with a certificate of registration and may use the initials I. S. Hom. You can contact the Society for the address of your local homeopath.

The following is a list of some of the menopause clinics — both National Health Service and private — in Ireland and the United Kingdom.

Ireland

Albany Women's Clinic
Clifton Court, Fitzwilliam Street Lower, Dublin 2.
Tel. 01 661 6029.

Coombe Hospital
Dolphin's Barn, Dublin 8. Tel. 01 453 7561.

Cork Family Planning Clinic
23 Tuckey Street, Cork. Tel. 021 277906.

Family Planning Services
67 Pembroke Road, Dublin 4. Tel. 01 668 3714.

Irish Family Planning Association
5 Cathal Brugha Street, Dublin 1. Tel. 01 872 7088.

Irish Family Planning Association
Level 3, The Square, Tallaght, Dublin 24. Tel. 01 459 7685.

Irish Family Planning Association
Synge Street Clinic, 59 Synge Street, Dublin 8. Tel. 01 478 0712.

Irish Family Planning Information Office
16 Lower O'Connell Street, Dublin 1. Tel. 01 878 0366.

National Maternity Hospital
Holles Street, Dublin 2. Tel. 01 661 0277.

Pembroke Clinic
34 Lower Pembroke Street, Dublin 2. Tel. 01 661 6610.

Rotunda Hospital
Parnell Square, Dublin 1. Tel. 01 873 0700.

Well Woman Clinic
73 Lower Leeson Street, Dublin 2. Tel. 01 661 0083.

Well Woman Clinic
35 Lower Liffey Street, Dublin 1. Tel. 01 872 8051.

Women's Medical Clinic
34 Main Street, Blackrock, Co. Dublin. Tel. 01 288 4943.

United Kingdom — NHS Clinies

Beckenham Hospital
379 Croydon Road, Beckenham, Kent CR3 3QL.
Tel. 0181 650 0125.

Birmingham and Midland Hospital for Women
Showell Green Lane, Sparkhill, Birmingham B11 4HL.
Tel. 0121 772 1101.

Birmingham Maternity Hospital
2nd Floor Clinic, Birmingham B15 2TG. Tel. 0121 472 1377.

City Hospital
Hucknall Road, Nottingham NG5 1TV. Tel. 0115 969 1169.

Dryburn Hospital
North Road, Durham DH1 5TW. Tel. 0191 386 4911.

Family Planning Clinic
18 Dean Terrace, Edinburgh EH4 1NL. Tel. 0131 332 7941.

Gavin Brown Clinic
Salthouse Road, Sutton, Hull HU8 9HE. Tel. 01482 701151.

Glasgow Royal Infirmary
85-86 Castle Street, Glasgow G4 0SF. Tel. 0141 552 3535.

Glasgow Western Infirmary
Dumbarton Road, Glasgow, G11 6NT. Tel. 0141 339 8822.

Guy's Hospital
St Thomas's Street, London SE1 9RT. Tel. 0171 955 5000.

Gynaecology Unit

Maternity Unit, Heath End Road, Nuneaton, Warwickshire CV10 7DJ. Tel. 01203 351351.

HRT Clinic

Caerphilly District, Miners Hospital, St Martin's Road, Caerphilly SF8 1WD. Tel. 01222 851811.

Hospital of St Cross

Barby Road, Rugby, Warwickshire CV22 5PX. Tel. 01788 572831.

John Radcliffe Hospital

Headington, Oxford OX3 9DU. Tel. 01865 741166.

Kings College Hospital

Denmark Hill, London SE5 9RS. Tel. 0171 274 6222.

Lewisham Hospital Menopause Clinic

A3 Ward, Second Floor, B Wing, Lewisham Hospital, Lewisham SE13 5LH. Tel. 0181 690 4311.

Margaret Pyke Centre

Soho Square, London W1V STW. Tel. 0171 734 9351.

Menopause Clinic

University Dept of Obstetrics and Gynaecology, Maternity Hospital, Cambridge CB2 5SW. Tel. 01223 336875.

Menopause Clinic

Gynaecology Department, Clarendon Wing, General Infirmary at Leeds, Belmont Grove, Leeds LS2 9NS. Tel. 01132 432799/437146.

Menopause Clinic
38 Walters Road, Swansea SA1 5 NW. Tel. 01792 655600.

Menopause Clinic
Singleton Hospital, Sketty, Swansea SA2 8QA.
Tel. 01792 205666.

Menopause Research Unit
Leicester Royal Infirmary, Infirmary Square, Leicester
LE1 5WW. Tel. 01162 523161.

Moor Street Clinic
Moor Street, Worcester WR1 3DB. Tel. 01905 21075.

Newcastle General Hospital
Westgate Road, Newcastle upon Tyne NE4 6BE.
Tel. 0191 273 8811.

Northern General Hospital
Gynaecology Department, Herries Road, Sheffield S5 7AU.
Tel. 0114 2434343.

Northwick Park Hospital
Watford Road, Harrow, Middlesex HA1 3UJ.
Tel. 0181 869 2863.

Postgraduate Centre
Anlaby Road, Hull. Tel. 01482 78541.

Princess Royal Hospital
Salthouse Road, Hull, North Humberside HU8 9HE.
Tel. 01482 701151.

Queen Charlotte's Hospital

Goldhawk Road, London W6 0XG. Tel. 0181 748 4666.

Royal Free Hospital

Pond Street, London NW3 2QG. Tel. 0171 794 0500.

Royal Liverpool Hospital

Catherine Street, Liverpool L8 7NJ. Tel. 0151 709 1000.

Royal Oldham Hospital

Menopause Clinic, Department of Obstetrics and
Gynaecology, Rochdale Road, Oldham, Lancashire OL1 2JH.
Tel. 0161 624 0420.

Samaritan Hospital for Women

Marylebone Road, London NW1 5UR. Tel. 0171 402 4211.

St George's Hospital

Blackshaw Road, London SW17 0QT. Tel. 0181 672 1255.

St Thomas's Hospital

Lambeth Palace Road, London SE1 7EH. Tel. 0171 928 9292.

Stafford District General Hospital

Weston Road, Stafford ST16 3SA. Tel. 01785 57731.

Stobhill Hospital

133 Balomock Road, Glasgow G21 3UW. Tel. 0141 558 0111.

Trafford Menopause Clinic

Chapel Road Clinic, Sale, Cheshire M33 1EG.
Tel. 0161 973 3415.

Well Woman Clinic
Alice Vieland Clinic, Bull Meadow Road, Exeter.
Tel. 01392 72741.

Women's Hospital
Gynaecological Clinic, Catherine Street, Liverpool L8 7NJ.
Tel. 0151 709 1000.

United Kingdom — Private Clinics

Amarant Trust
80 Lambeth Road, London SE1 7PW. Tel. 0171 401 3855.

Beeches Consulting Centre
Mill Lane, Cheadle, Cheshire SK8 2PY. Tel. 0161 491 2606.

BUPA Medical Centre
(Well Woman Screening Clinic), Battle Bridge House, 300
Gray's Inn Road, London WC1X 8DU. Tel. 0171 837 6484.

Haslemere House
68 Haslemere Avenue, Mitcham, Surrey. Tel. 0181 648 3234.

Highfield Clinic
Highfield Lane, St Albans, Hertfordshire AL4 0RJ.
Tel. 01727 44777.

Nuffield Hospital Health Screening Unit
Clayton Road, Jesmond, Newcastle upon Tyne NE2 1JP.
Tel. 0191 281 6131.

Richmond Hill Clinic (Brook Advisory Centre)
25-27 Denmark Street, Bristol BS1 5DQ.
Tel. 0117 929 2136.

St John's Medical Centre
St John's Road, Altrincham, Cheshire WA14 2NW.
Tel. 0161 928 8727.

Well Woman Centre
Marie Stopes House, 108 Whitfield Street, London W1P 6BE.
Tel. 0171 388 0662.

8 Devonshire Place, London W1N 1PB. Tel. 0171 935 2357.

9a Wilbraham Place, Sloane Street, London S1X 9AE.
Tel. 0171 730 7928.

12 Thurloe Street, London SW7 2SP. Tel. 0171 584 6204.

20 Church Road, Edgbaston, Birmingham B15 3TA.
Tel. 0121 454 2345.

25 Britannia Pavilion, Albert Dock, Liverpool L3 4AA.
Tel. 0151 709 3998.

31 Rodney Street, Liverpool L1 9EH. Tel. 0151 709 8522.

56 Harley Street, London W1N 1AE. Tel. 0171 580 6332.

120 Harley Street, London W1N 1AG, Tel. 0171 486 0497.

886 Garratt Lane, London SW17. Tel. 0181 672 1948.

Sources of Natural Progesterone

Halmont Ltd
Sidmonton Avenue, Bray, Co. Wicklow. Tel. 01 286 6280.

Health Ministry
The Nutrition Centre, Donegal Town, Co. Donegal.

Natural Healing Rooms
8 Wolfe Tone Street, Clonakilty, Co. Cork. Tel. 023 34748.

Further Reading

Achterberg, Jeanne, *Woman as Healer*, Massachusetts: Shambhala 1990.

Assilem, Melissa, *Women Ripening through the Menopause*, California: Idolatry Ink 1996.

Grof, Stanislav, and Christina Grof, *The Stormy Search for the Self*, Mandala 1991.

Kenton, Leslie, *Passage to Power*, London: Ebury Press 1995.

Lee, John R., *Natural Progesterone: The Multiple Roles of a Remarkable Hormone*, California: BLL Publishing 1993.

Lee, John R., *Optimal Health Guidelines*, California: BLL Publishing 1994.

Northrup, Christiane, *Women's Bodies, Women's Wisdom*, New York: Bantam Books 1994.

Pinkola Estes, Clarissa, *Women Who Run With the Wolves*, London: Rider 1992.

Reitz, Rosetta, *Menopause, a Positive Approach*, London: Unwin Paperbacks 1985.

Vines, Gail, *Raging Hormones*, London: Virago 1993.

What Doctor's Don't Tell You Limited, *Guide to the Menopause*, London: The Wallace Press 1997.

Index